ENTRANCE EXAMINATION IN RHEUMATOLOGY

(Includes Important Text, MCQ's with Explanations)

Editor :
Dr. M.S. Bhatia (M.D.; MNAMS)
Prof & Head, Department of Psychiatry
University College of Medical Sciences &
Guru Teg Bahadur Hospital,
Dilshad Garden Delhi - 110095,

Contributing Editor :
Dr. (Mrs.) Nirmaljit Kaur (M.D.)
Senior Specialist, Department of Microbiology
Dr. R.M.L., Hospital
New Delhi - 110001

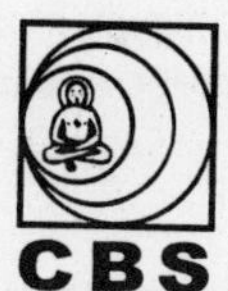

CBS PUBLISHERS & DISTRIBUTORS PVT. LTD.
New Delhi • Bangalore • Pune • Cochin • Chennai (India)

ISBN : 978-81-239-2220-1

First Edition : 2012

Published by Satish Kumar Jain and produced by V.K. Jain for
CBS Publishers & Distributors Pvt. Ltd.,
CBS Plaza, 4819/XI Prahlad Street, 24 Ansari Road, Daryaganj,
New Delhi - 110002, India. • Website: www.cbspd.com
e-mail: delhi@cbspd.com, cbspubs@airtelmail.in
Ph.: 23289259, 23266861, 23266867 • Fax: 011-23243014

Branches:

- ***Bengaluru:*** Seema House, 2975, 17th Cross, K.R. Road,
  Bansankari 2nd Stage, Bengaluru - 560070
  • Ph.: +91-80-26771678/79 • Fax: +91-80-26771680
  • E-mail: cbsbng@gmail.com, bangalore@cbspd.com
- ***Pune:*** Bhuruk Prestige, Sr. No. 52/12/2+1+3/2,
  Narhe, Haveli (Near Katraj-Dehu Road By-pass), Pune - 411051
  • Ph.: +91-20-64704058/59, 32342277 • E-mail: pune@cbspd.com
- ***Kochi:*** 36/14, Kalluvilakam, Lissie Hospital Road,
  Kochi - 682018, Kerala • Ph.: +91-484-4059061-65
  • Fax: +91-484-4059065 • E-mail: cochin@cbspd.com
- ***Chennai:*** 20, West Park Road, Shenoy Nagar, Chennai - 600030
  Ph.: +91-44-26260666, 26208620 • Fax: +91-44-42032115
  • E-mail: chennai@cbspd.com

Printed at :
J.S. Offset Printers, Delhi

Dedicated to our Parents

&

beloved Children

PREFACE

Medical science is a rapidly advancing field. Its new allied branches are coming up. In a competitive examination, more and more emphasis is being laid on these allied disciplines. But most of the standard textbooks of medicine have failed to devote adequate space to these new disciplines.

This book has been written with the aim to outline the major areas of Rheumatology, a new superspeciality. This book is not merely an addition to the existing list of books on MCQ's but a sincere ambition and an honest attempt to make it a useful and practical companion to both medical graduates and postgraduates. The present book consists of original solved MCQ's from the *Question Banks* of various important examinations (AIIMS, Delhi, PGI etc.), Important text, original solved MCQ's and their explanations have been added. We hope that this will help the candidates in performing better in the examination.

All suggestions for the modification of this book are welcome and will be duly acknowledged.

—Editors

CONTENTS

IMPORTANT TEXT

INTRODUCTION

RHEUMATISM

Rheumatism is a non-specific term used to describe many painful disorder affecting the loco-motor system including joints, muscles, connective tissues, soft tissues around the joints and bones. The term rheumatism is also used to describe rheumatic fever affecting heart valves. However, the medical profession uses specific terms to describe rheumatological disorders such as rheumatoid arthritis, ankylosing spondylitis, gout and systemic lupus erythematosus and so on in the medical literature.

Rheumatology is now emerging as an important clinical speciality recognized all over the world. The speciality is rapidly improving and well established along with properly organized post graduate training programs. The term describing clinicians dealing with rheumatism as "***rheumatologists***" is now a well established term commonly used by the medical community, even though it is not adequately described in dictionaries established for languages. Rheumatologists all over the world are now capable of treating most of the chronic rheumatological disorders with much better outcome for the patients. This is due to the discovery of new disease modifying agents called biologics which is now a well established form of treatment for the patients suffering from chronic and disabling joint disorders.

RHEUMATOLOGIST

A rheumatologist is a physician specialized in the field of medical sub-speciality called rheumatology, and holds either a board certification after specialized training after Doctor of Medicine Degree or has DM in India or equivalent programs elsewhere in the world. In the United States, training in this field requires four years undergraduate of medical school, and then three years of residency, followed by two or three years additional Fellowship training. The number of years allocated for specialized training in rheumatology for postgraduate trainees in different countries could vary according to the requirements of different countries.

Rheumatologists treat arthritis, certain autoimmune disease, musculoskeletal pain disorders and osteoporosis. There are more than 200 types of these diseases, including rheumatoid arthritis, osteoarthritis, gout, lupus, back pain, osteoporosis, and tendinitis. They treat soft tissue problems related to musculoskeletal system, sports related soft tissue disorders and the specialty is also inter-related with physiotherapy, physical medicine and rehabilitation.

There are many international organizations representing rheumatologists all over the world. The American College of Rheumatology (ACR), the Association of Rheumatology Health Professionals (ARHP), the European League Against Rheumatism (EULAR), Asia Pacific League of Associations for Rheumatology (APLAR), International League of Associations for Rheumatology (ILAR) and the British Society of Rheumatology (BSR) are the main international organizations established and organizing many activities related to this speciality.

Degenerative arthropathies

* Osteoarthritis
* Inflammatory arthropathies
* Rheumatoid arthritis
* Spondyloarthropathies
  * Ankylosing spondylitis
  * Reactive arthritis (reactive arthropathy)
  * Psoriatic arthropathy
  * Enteropathic spondylitis
* Juvenile Idiopathic Arthritis (JIA)
* Crystal arthropathies : gout, pseudogout
* Septic arthritis
* Ross river virus
* Barmah forest virus

Systemic conditions and connective tissue diseases

* Lupus
* Sjogren's syndrome
* Scleroderma (systemic sclerosis)
* Polymyositis

* Dermatomyositis
* Polymyalgia rheumatica
* Mixed connective tissue disease
* Polychondritis
* Sarcoidosis
* Vasculitis
* Polyarteritis nodosa
* Henoch-Schonlein purpura
* Serum sickness
* Wegener's granulomatosis
* Giant cell arteritis, Temporal arteritis
* Takayasu's arteritis
* Behcet's syndrome
* Kawasaki's disease (mucocutaneous lymph node syndrome)
* Buerger's disease (thromboangiitis obliterans)

Soft Tissue Rheumatism

* Low back pain
* Tennis elbow
* Golfer's elbow
* Olecranon bursitis

Fibromyalgia

Diseases affecting bones

* Osteoporosis
* Osteomalacia
* Renal osteodystrophy
* Fluorosis
* Rickets

Congenital and familial disorders affecting joints

* Hyperextensible joints
* Ehlers-Danlos syndrome
* Achondroplasia
* Marfan's syndrome

IMPORTANT TEXT OF RHEUMATOLOGY

IMPORTANT POINTS

* The commonest chronic inflammatory joint disease - Rheumatoid Arthritis (RA).
* The age incidence of Rheumatoid Arthritis is 20 to 50 years.
* The most commonly susceptible HLA group in Rheumatoid arthritis is DR4.
* In India, the HLA susceptible to RA is DR1.
* The basic pathological mechanism in RA is T-cell activation.
* The earliest change in RA - swelling of synovial membrane.
* **Swindled appearance** of hands is seen in RA
* Rheumatoid factors are immunoglobulins of the class IgG, IgM.
* The most sensitive tests for RA are **Nephelometric** tests.
* Incidence of positive **Rose-Waaler** test in patients of RA is 70%.
* The screening test for RA is latex fixation test.
* The drug used for intra-articular injections in RA is Methyl prednisolone.
* Anti-TB drug used for RA is Captopril.
* Anti-hypertensive drug used for RA is Prednisolone
* Antithelminthic drug used in RA is Levimasole.
* Medical synovectomy for large joints is with **yitrium** 90 silicate.
* Medical synovectomy for small joints is with **erbium** 159 acetate.
* Extra-articular manifestations in RA indicate bad prognosis
* Artificial tears used in sjogren's syndrome contain Hypromellose.

* Proportion of patients of RA achieving remission after splenectomy is 60%.
* Ankylosing spondylitis has a predilection to sacroiliac joints.
* Rheumatic disease associated with inflammatory bowel disease is ankylosing spondylitis.
* The characteristic pathologicla lesion in ankylosing spondylitis is **Enthesopathy**
* The new bone formation in ankylosing spondylitis - Syndesmophyte.
* Rheumatic disease causing chest pain increasing during breathing is Ankylosing spondylitis.
* The commonest extraarticular manifestation of ankylosing spondylitis is uveitis.
* The male to female ratio in ankylosing spondylitis is 50%.
* Keratoderma blenorrhagica is a feature of reiter's syndrome.
* Arthritis **mutilans** in psoriatic arthropathy indicates bad prognosis.
* The most common pattern of psoriatic arthropathy is assymetrical oligoarthritis.
* The inflammatory bowel disease in which enteropathic synovitis is most common - Crohn's disease.
* Exception to Aspirin contraindication in children below 12 years - Juvenile chronica arthritis.
* The commonest cause of septic arthritis in Infancy - Hemophilus influenzae.
* **"Rubbed out"** appearance of joints is seen in - Septic Arthritis.
* **"Erythema chronicum migrans"** is the rash seen in Lyme Arthritis.
* Causative organism of lyme fever is Borrelia burghdorferi.
* Fungal infections associated with Erythema nodosum - Histoplasmosis, Coccidiodomycosis.
* Proportion of patients of Hepatitis B, developing Arthritis is 40%.
* Time interval between the appearance of rash and onset of Arthritis in Rubella is 1 to 7 days.

* Granulomatous disease causing punched out lesions - Sarcoidosis.
* Commonest presenting features of systemic lupus erythmatosis (SLE) - Arthralgia with fever.
* Commonest mode of onset of Rheumatoid Arthritis (RA) - Palindromic.
* **"Chilblain' like lesions** are seen in - SLE.
* Bullous eruptions and panniculitis are known as - lupus profundus.
* Proportion of patients of SLE having Alopecia is 50%.
* **"Shrinking lung syndrome"** is a feature of SLE.
* The prominent cardiac manifestation of SLE is **Libman sachs** Endocarditis.
* Gastrointestinal complication of corticosteroid therapy in SLE is Gastric and Duodenal perforation.
* Abdominal mass in patients of SLE is due to splenomegaly.
* 5 years survival in patients with SLE is 90%.
* **"Sausage swelling"** of fingers is seen in systemic sclerosis.
* **"Mask face"** and **"Beak nose"** are features of Scleroderma.
* **Heliotrope rash** on upper eyelids is seen in Dermatomyositis.
* The inheritance of Lesch Nyhan syndrome is - X-linked recessive.
* The enzyme defect in Lesch Nyhan syndrome is **HGPRTase** deficiency".
* **Chronic fatigue syndrome** is due to myalgic encephalitis.
* The inheritance of achondroplasia is Autosomal dominant.
* The height of adult achondroplasiac is less than 4'3".
* Facial features in achondroplasia - Large head, bulging forehead, Depressed nasal bridge.
* **Trident hand** is a feature of - achondroplasia.
* The lateral diameter of pelvis is increased in Achondroplasia.
* Spinal canal is narrowed in the anteroposterior diameter in Achondroplasia.
* Osteogenesis imperfecta is also known as **Fragilitas ossium**.

* Inheritance of osteogenesis imperfecta - Autosomal dominant.
* Auditory association with osteogenesis imperfecta - Otosclerosis.
* Osteochondroma in diaphyseal aclasis form at Metaphysis.
* Malignancy that occurs in diaphyseal aclasis - Chondrosarcoma.
* Multiple enchondromatosis is also known as Ollier's disease.
* Paget's disease is literally absent in India.
* **Commonest** site for Paget's disease - Pelvis, next vertebra.
* Age incidence of Paget's disease - above 40 years.
* Enzyme marker for Paget's disease - Alkaline phosphatase.
* **Most common** complication of Paget's disease - Pathological fracture.
* **Drug of choice** for Paget's disease - Diphosphonates.
* **Commonest** bone affected in polyostotic fibrous dysplasia - Femur.
* Ground glass appearance on X-ray is a feature of Polyostatic fibrous dysplasia.
* Albright's syndrome constitutes :
  - **Polyostotic** fibrous dysplasia
  - Skin pigmentation
  - Precocity in females
* The inheritance of Neurofibromatosis - Autosomal dominant.
* **Commonest** pathological **fracture** in neurofibromatosis is of Tibia.
* Microdactyly is a feature of Myositis ossificans progressiva.
* Inheritance of myositis ossificans progressiva - Autosomal dominant.
* **Most striking feature** of craniocleido dystosis - Enlargement of frontal and parietal bones.
* The inheritance of Gaucher's disease is Autosomal.
* Enzyme defect in Gaucher's disease - β glucuronidase.
* Substance accumulating in Gaucher's disease - Glucocerebroside.
* Gaucher cells are - Lipid laden reticuloendothelial cells.

* **Forms of Histiocytosis-X**
  - Letterer-Siwe disease
  - Hand-Schuller-Christian disease
  - Eosinophilic granuloma
* **Most serious form** of histocytosis X - Letterer Siwe disease.
* **Cupping of metaphysis** of bones is a feature of Rickets.
* Familial hypophosphatemia is also known as Chronic phosphate diabetes.
* Familial hypophosphatemia is inherited as X-linked dominant.
* **Looser's zones** - feature of osteomalacia.
* **Looser's zones** are - Multiple spontaneous fractures.
* Vitamin deficiency causing **pseudoparalysis** - Vitamin C.
* Skeletal features of Scurvy in Infants resemble - Syphilitic metaphysitis.
* Close differential diagnosis for scurvy - Osteomyelitis.
* Prevention of osteoporosis in postmenopausal woman is by Estrogen
* Sympathetic effusion is a feature of Osteomyelitis.
* **Complications of osteomyelitis** :
  - Septicemia
  - Pyogenic arthritis
  - Decreased growth
* Drug of choice for acute osteomyelitis - Flucloxacillin.
* Devitalised area in acute osteomyelitis - Sequestrum.
* New bone formation in acute osteomyelitis - Involucrum.
* **Honey combed** appearance is a feature of - Chronic osteomylitis.
* Systemic disease complicating chronic osteomyelitis - Amyloidosis.
* **Brodie's abscess** is usually situated at Metaphysis.
* Predominat symptoms of Brodie's abscess - Deep boring pain.
* Radiologically, Brodie's abscess appears as Round cavity surrounded by a zone of sclerosis.

* Hodgkin's disease causes osteolytic lesions.
* Close differential diagnosis for simple bone cyst - Bone abscess.
* Endocrine disorder causing simple bone cyst - Hyperparathyroidism.
* The nidus in osteoid osteoma forms in Cortex.
* Close differential diagnosis for osteoid osteoma - Brodie's abscess.
* Polymyalgia rheumatica usually affects - Woman above 60 years.
* Polymyalgia rheumatica is associated with giant cell arteritis.
* Drug of choice in polymyalgia rheumatica - Prednisolone.
* **Common causative organisms of pyogenic arthritis :**
  - Staphylococcus (Commonest)
  - Streptococcus
  - Penumococcus
  - Salmonella
* Peripheral joints are commonly affected in Rheumatoid Arthritis (RA).
* Clinical features of RA are more severe in - Seropositive patients.
* The seronegative arthritis may be associated with - Osteoarthritis (OA).
* Most commonly affected joints in TB arthritis - Spine.
* **Earliest** radiological change in TB arthritis - Diffuse rarefaction.
* **Complications of TB Arthritis** - Sinus formations.
  - Secondary infection
  - Spread to another part
* **Predisposing factors to osteoarthritis :**
  - Congenital development
  - Malunion
  - Previous fracture
  - Obesity
  - Rheumatoid arthritis
* Coarse crepitus during movement is a feature of Osteo arthritis (OA).
* **Radiological features of OA** - Decreased cartilage space
  - Subchondral sclerosis
  - Osteophyte formation

* The crystals deposited in Gout - monosodium urate monohydrate.
* The first attack of gout is usually in the first toe.
* Bursa most often affected by gout - Olecranon bursa.
* Definitive treatment for synovial chondromatosis - Subtotal synovectomy.
* Erb's palsy - Injury to upper roots of brachial plexus (C5,6).
* Klumpke palsy - injury to lower roots of Brachial Plexus (C8, T1).
* Prognosis is better in Erb's palsy.
* **Commonest** cause of brachial plexus injuries in adults - Motorcycling accidents.
* Sternomastoid tumour - Infantile torticollis (Earliest swelling in infancy).
* Surgery for sternomastoid tumour - von **Lockum's** operation.
* Congenital high scapula - Sprengel's shoulder.
* Cervical spondylosis, is **most common** in the lower three cervical vertebrae.
* The changes of cervical spondylosis first affect the - Central Intervertebral joints.
* A cervical rib develops from - Costal process of C7.
* Close differential diagnosis for scalenus syndrome - Prolapse of C7 and T1.
* **Straight leg raising test** is positive in sciatica.
* **Most common** type of scoliosis - Idiopathic.
* Onset of idiopathic scoliosis - 10 to 12 years.
* **Milwaukee brace** is used for childhood scoliosis.
* **Milwaukee brace** employs the method of 3 point correction.
* Correction of scoliosis at surgery is by - **Harrington** distraction rod.
* Common causes of secondary structural scoliosis.
  - Hemivertebra
  - Poliomyelitis
  - Neurofibromatosis

* Temporary scoliosis - Sciatic scoliosis
* Sciatic scoliosis is produced by - Protective muscle spasm
* **Commonest** underlying cause for sciatic scoliosis - Prolapsed disc.
* The infection in Pott's spine begins at - Anterior margin of vertebra.
* Commonest cold abscess in Pott's spine psoas abscess.
* Psoas abscess usually points in the Iliac fossa.
* Neurological manifestation of Pott's spine - Paraplegia
* OA of the spine - Spondyloarthritis.
* Ankylosing spondylitis is also known as - **Marie Strumpell disease.**
* Poker back is a feature of Ankylosing spondylitis.
* Earliest X-ray feature of Ankylosing spondylitis - Iridocyclitis.
* Ophthalmic complication of Ankylosing spondylitis - Iridocyclitis.
* Adolescent kyphosis is known as - **Scheurman's disease.**
* **Commonest** site of Disc prolapse - Lumbar.
* The nucleus palposus protrudes through the posteriolateral part.
* Spontaneous displacement of vertebral body - Spondylolisthesis.
* Definitive treatment for RA of shoulder - Replacement Arthroplasty.
* The pain in **supraspinatus syndrome** occurs during 45 - 160 degrees movement.
* Initiation of Abduction is impaired in torn supraspinatus syndrome.
* Acromioclavicular arthritis mimics supraspinatus syndrome closely.
* **Yagarson's sign** is diagnostic of Biceps tendinitis.
* Cubitus valgus predisposis to friction neuritis of ulnar nerve
* **Commonest** cause of cubitus valgus - Fracture lower end Humerus with malunion.
* Usual number of loose bodies in synovial chondromatosis - **50 to 500.**

* **Tardy ulnar palsy** is a feature of Cubitus valgus.
* The deviation in RA wrist and hand - **Ulnar drift.**
* **Heberden's nodes** is a feature of OA of interphalangeal pints.
* Finger pulp space infection is also known as - whitlow felon.
* **Honey comb finger** is a feature of - Felon
* **Commonest** cause of chronic infective tenosynovitis - TB.
* **Phalen's test** is diagnostic of - Carpal tunnel syndrome.
* In carpal tunnel syndrome, the median nerve is compressed against the flexor retinaculum.
* **Tinel's sign** is seen in - Carpal tunnel syndrome.
* **Commonest** cystic swelling at the back of neck - Ganglion.
* Deformity in Dupuytren's contracture starts in the Ring finger, and is limited to ring and little fingers.
* Avulsion of extensor tendon from Distal phalanx - Mallet/ Baseball finger.
* Tenovaginitis of Abductor pollucis and Extensor pollucis brevis - dequervain's tenovaginitis.
* Digital tenovaginitis stenosans - Trigger finger.
* Method of reduction of congenital dislocation of Hip - Barlow's manoeuvre.
* **Surgeries of congenital dislocation of Hip (CDH) :**
  - Salter's operation
  - Pemberton's operation
  - Wainwright's operation
  - Chiari's operation
* Pyogenic arthritis in infants - Tom Smith's disease.
* **Common** arthritis in Hip - TB arthritis.
* Earliest radiological feature of TB Hip - Diffuse rarefaction.
* Radio-isotope scan in Perthe's disease shows - failure of uptake. Most other diseases show increased uptake.
* Perthe's disease may predispose to OA.

* Slipped upper femoral epiphysis predisposes to OA.
* Movements limited in coxa vera - flexion, abduction and medial rotation.
* The neck shaft angle in Coxa vera - Osteotomy below greater trochanter.
* **Lachman's test** is for anterior and posterior cruciate ligaments.
* **Mc Murray's test** is for - tears of meniscus.
* Tumours metastasising to Bone - Lung, Breast, Prostate, Kidney, Thyroid.
* **Commonest** site for pyogenic arthritis - Knee.
* **Commonest** site for OA - Knee.
* **Commonest** site of Hemarthrosis - Knee.
* **Commonest** predisposing factor for OA - Overweight.
* **First feature** of OA of Knee - Sharping/spiking joints.
* Course of OS good Schlatter's disease - self-limiting.
* Herniation of synovial cavity of knee - **Baker's cyst.**
* Normal dorsiflexion of big toe is 90 degrees.
* Commonest congenital deformity of foot - congenital talipes equinovarus (CTEV).
* Crucial component of deformity of CTEV- Subluxation of Talonavicular joint.
* Components of deformity of CTEV - Inversion, Adduction, Equinus contracture.
* The components of CTEV corrected first - Adduction, Inversion.
* **Hollow feet** - pes cavus.
* Surgery for pes cavus - Steindler muscle slide operation.
* **Kohler's disease** is confined to children between 3 to 5 years of age.
* **Phenolisation** is done for ingrowing toe nail.
* Definitive treatment for ingrowing toe nail - Excision of germinal matrix.

ALTERNATE NAMES OF DISEASE

1.	Apophysitis of Tibial Tubercle	-	Osgood Schlatter disease
2.	Apophysitis of Calcaneus	-	Sever's disease
3.	Osteochondritis of Navicular bone	-	Kohler's disease
4.	Osteochondritis of Lunate bone	-	Keinbock's disease
5.	Osteochondritis of Femoral head Epiphyses	-	Perthe's disease
6.	Osteochondritis dissecans of Metatarsal head	-	Freiberg disease
7.	Radioulnar dyschondro-osteosis	-	Madelung deformity
8.	Prepatellar bursitis	-	Housemaid's knee
9.	Suprapatellar bursitis	-	Clergyman's knee
10.	Traumatic olecranon bursitis	-	Student's elbow
11.	Avulsion of extensor tendons of Forearm	-	Tennis elbow
12.	Avulsion of Flexor tendons of Forearm	-	Golfer's elbow
13.	Multiple synovial chondromatosis	-	Ollier's disease
14.	Plantar digital neuritis	-	Morton's metatarsalgia
15.	Avulsion of extensor tendon of distal phalynx	-	Mallet/Baseball finger
16.	Digital tenovaginitis stenosans	-	Trigger finger
17.	Pyogenic Arthritis in infants	-	Tomsmith's disease
18.	Adolescent kyphosis	-	Scheurman's disease
19.	Ankylosing spondylitis	-	Marie strumpell arthritis
20.	Vertical fracture distal end of Radius	-	Barton's fracture
21.	Fracture 1st metacarpal with carpometacarpal dislocation	-	Bennet's fracture
22.	Fracture upper 1/3 of Ulna	-	Monteggia fracture dislocation with head of radius

ALTERNATE NAMES OF DISEASE (Contd...)

23.	Lower 1/3 of Radius fracture with dislocation of inferior radioulnar joint	-	Galezzi fracture dislocation
24.	Fracture lower end radius with Ulnar styloid process	-	Colles fracture
25.	Reversed Colles fracture	-	Smith's fracture
26.	Sub ligamentous hematoma after avulsion of medial ligament of knee	-	Pallegrini stieda's disease

SOME NAMED TESTS, SIGNS & OPERATIONS

1. Jactitation - Intermittent spasm of amputation stump
2. Birgess amputation - Below knee with long posterior flap
3. Pirogoff's amputation - Modification of syme
4. Chopart's amputation - Through midtarsal joint
5. Lisfrance's amputation - Through tarsometatarsal joint
6. Krukenberg's amputation - Forearm bones amputated, and bones used as a fork for gripping
7. Guillotone amputation - Emergency amputation in gas - gangrene
8. Hindquarter amputation - Removal of LL with often, ischium, pubis.
9. Crammer wire is a splint.
10. Duration between traumatic amputation & reimplatation - within 10 hours.
11. Pollicization - Transplantation of finger to provide thumb.
12. Campbell's operation - For poliomyelitis.
13. Soutter's operation - For flexor contracture of hip.
14. Vitlium - alloy of Cd, Ni, Mb (cadmium, nickel, molybdnum).
15. Position of eye of IM nail during nailing - posteromedial.
16. Nobman Rowe disimpaction forceps - used to disrupt zygomatic process of maxilla fracture.

17. Charlie Chaplin gait - Tibial torsion
18. Skew foot - congenital metatarsus adductovarus.
19. Russels traction for - Juvenile RA
20. Gee's disease - celiac disease
21. Jungling's disease - Sarcoidosis
22. Mitten hand - Removal of all fingers & thumb
23. Ullmans sign (X-ray) - spondylolisthesis
24. Slocum test - Anterolateral instability of knee.
25. Chin on chest deformity. Ankylosing spondylitis.
26. Tonton kells - Histocytosis
27. Step sign +ve in - Spondylolisthesis
    - Acromioclavicular dislocation
28. China blue sclerosis - Fragilitis ossium.
29. Slate blue sclerosis - Ochronosis.
30. Cock-up deformity - Diebetic neuropathy of Tibial nerve.
31. Tumour albus - TB arthritis
32. Muscle called peripheral heart - Soleus.
33. Miners beat knee - Acute suppurative prepatellar bursitis.
34. Fimmounts test - Complete rupture of Achilles tendon.
35. Cinema Sign - Primary adolescent chondromalacia patella.
36. Fish net traction - Scoliosis
37. Q-angle - Recurrent dislocation of patella
38. Coins test - Pott's spine
39. Christian triad
    - Defect in membranous bones
    - Exophthalmos
    - DI
40. Frog position - Acute suppurative arthritis of hip.
41. Oath Hand - High median nerve palsy.
42. Thomsons test - To detect rupture of Tendoachilles.
43. In Tennis leg, gastrocnemius is invariably ruptured.

44. Earliest lab finding in fat embolism - lipemia.
45. Boxers fracture - Fracture neck of 4th or 5th metacarpal.
46. Chauffer's fracture - Transverse fracture LE radius extending laterally from articular surface.
47. Saturday night fracture - fracture neck of 5th metacarpal.
48. Hume fracture - proximal ulna fracture + Radial dislocation in children.
49. Talwaker square nail used for - fracture Radius or ulna.
50. **Commonest** nerve to be injured in galaezzi fracture dislocation - Ulnar nerve.
51. Hamilton ruler test - Anterior dislocation of shoulder.
52. Jones strapping (3 wk) - Acromioclavicular dislocation.
53. Naffjigher's test - lumbar disc prolapse.
54. Porter's shoulder - Adventious bursa between superior surface of clavicle & skin.
55. Golder's shoulder - Biceps Tendinitis - Yagarson's test.
56. Tennis elbow - Avulsion of lower extensor origin
57. Golfer's elbow - Avulsion of lower flexor origin.
58. Student's Miner's elbow - Subluxation of proximal radioulnar joint.
59. Nurse maid elbow - subluxation of proximal radioulnar joint.
60. Baseball pithcer elbow - Hyper trophy of Humerus - Humerus no longer fits in the olecranon fossa.
61. Little leaguers elbow - Variant of baseball pitchers elbow in children.
62. Jauveline elbow - Pain at triceps insertion.
63. Elbow Tunnel syndrome - ulnar nerve affected between the two heads of FCV.
64. Dequervain's disease - stenosing tenovaginitis of APB & FPB.
    * Trigger finger - digital stenosing tenovaginitis of flexor tendons of finger.
    * Trigger thumb - stenosing tenovaginitis of FPL.
65. ELBEES interspinous grafing - Potts paraplegia.

66. Charnley's compression arthrodesis - TB ankle joint
   * TB shoulder joint starts in UE humerus.
   * Melon seed bodies - TB tensynovitis, compound palmar ganglion.
   * Rotator cuff muscles - Subscapularis, supraspinatus infrapinatus, Teres minor.

67 Mill's test - Tennis elbow
   * Wadding gait - Bilateral CDH, bilateral coxa vera
   * Waldenstrom figure - Perthes, disease

68. PODAGRA - 1st metatarosophalangealgeal joint involved in gout.
   * Pencil in cup deformity of interphalangeal joints - psoriasis.
   * **Order of fusion of epiphysis at elbow**

     C-Capitulum 3 y

     I—Internal epicondyle 6 y

     T—Trochlea 9y

     E—External epicondyle 12 y
   * Shenton' line (upper border of obturator foramen to lower neck of femur) is distracted in :

   P—Perthes, disease

   T—TB arthritis hip

   C—CDH
   * Posterior dislocation of hip : attitude-flexion, adduction, and internal rotation (FAIR).
   * Anterior dislocation of hip : attitude-flexion, abduction and external rotation (FABEX) (PDH) Bryants vertical line shorted, cross-line lengthened.
   * RA can involve any joint except sacroiliac joint.
   * Ankylosis : NEVER occurs in OA
   * Ankylosing : spondylitis most commonly involves sacroiliac joint.

* Dowagiers hump - senile osteoporosis
* Dupuytren's contracture associated with :
   - Alcoholic cirrhosis - Stroke
   - Peyronie's disease of penis - phenytoin
   - Pallegrini Steidas disease

* **Scurvy :**
  - Wimburger's sign
  - White line of Frenkel
  - Trumerfeld zone
* **Barton's disease**

  (Scurvy rickets) combined deficiency of vit.C & D.
* Game keepers thumb - rupture of medial collateral ligament of metacarpophalangeal joint.
* Hook sign - whitlow
* Most serious infection of hand - infection of ulnar bursa
* Traumatic flat foot - collapse of longitudinal arch
* Pes cavus
  - Fredriech's ataxia
  - Poliomyelitis
  - Idiopathic
* Weavers bottom - between gluteus maximum & ischial tuberosity.
* Parrots pseudoparalysis - Early congenital syphilis
* Snow storm appearance
  - Synovial sarcoma (bone)
  - Fat embolism
  - Hydatidiform mole
  - Histiocytosis
* All being tumors except osteoid osteoma & osteoclastoma stop growing on skeletal maturity.
* **Osteoclastoma**
  - Indistinguishable from Brown tumours of Hyperparathyroidism.
  - Egg shell crackling on palpation
  - Soap-bubble appearance.
* **Multiple myeloma**
  - Vertebra is the commonest site
  - 45 - 65 y
  - Amyloid formation (AA)
  - Seive skull
  - M-spike

* **Most common** cause of Bone secondaries - Ca breast
  Next - Ca. prostate
* **Most common** presenting feature of bone secondaries - pain
* **Diaphyseal tumours**
  - Ewings sarcoma
  - Adamantinoma
  - Enchondroma
* **Hemangioma**
  - Site vertebra
  - Disappearing tumour of bone
  - Paraplegia
  - Phantom bone tumour

HLA-ASSOCIATED RHEUMATIC DISEASES

Disease	HLA Antigen
* Ankylosing spondylitis	B 27
* Reiter's syndrome	B27
* Reactive arthritis (Yersinia, Salmonella, Shigella)	B27
* Psoriatic arthritis	
* Peripheral	Bw38, Bw39
* Spondylitis	B27
* Inflammatory bowel disease	
* Spondylitis	B27
* Rheumatoid arthritis (adult)	DR4, DR1
* Juvenile arthritis	
* Seropositive, Polyarticular	DR4
* Pauciarticular	DR5, Dw5, DRw8, Dw52, Dpw2, Drw6
* Spondylitis	B27
* Still's disease	Bw35, DR4
* Systemic lupus erythematosus	**DR3, DR2, DQw1**
* With SS-A (Ro)	DR3
* With C2 deficiency	DR2 (Dw2), A25, B18

* Subacute cutaneous lupus erythematosus	DR3
* Drug-induced lupus erythematosus	DR4
* Sjogren's syndrome	
* Primary	DR2, DR3, DRw52
* With rheumatoid arthritis	DR4, DRw52, DRW53
* With systemic lupus erythematosus	DR3, Dqw1/DQw2, DRw52
* Polymysositis	
* Caucasians	DR3
* Blacks	DRw6
* Jo-1 positive	Dr3, Drw6
* Childhood	B8, Dr3
* Scleroderma	
* CREST	DR6
* Anticentromere positive	DR1

SYNDROMES

* **Behcet's syndrome :**
    * Unknown etiology
* Recurrent attacks of painful genital ulcerations.
* Asymmetrical polyarticular arthritis, Uveitis, hypopyon retinitis.
* Ulcerative skin lesions, erythema nodosum, thrombophlebitis.
* Encephalitis, convulsions, CN palsies, spinal cord and brain stem lesions.
* Characterised by remissions and exacerbations.
* **Crest syndrome :**
* Scleroderma (benign type)
  — Calcinosis (subcutaneous), Raynaud's phenomenon, collagen disorders, sclerodactyly. Telangiectasia of face, oral mucosa and hands.
* **Felty's syndrome :**
  Long standing cases of SLE and RA
  — Splenomegaly, chronic leucopenia, thrombocytopenia and anaemia.

* **Reiter's syndrome :**
  - — Urethritis, conjunctivitis, bilateral arthritis and muco-cutaneous lesions on glans penis, mouth, palms and soles. (Keratoderma blennorrhagia). Most patients settle spontaneously in 4-6 wks. Recurrent attacks may occur.

    Treatment : Support with mydriatics and local steroids for iritis.
* **Sjogren's syndrome : (AR)**

  (Sicca syndrome)
  - — Exclusively in females, failure of adequate secretions of mucous glands. Dryness of mouth and mucosmembrane dysphagia, painful swelling of joints. Alopecia, purpura, deficiency of lacrimation leads to drying of corners, conjunctiva, keratoconjunctivitis.

CLASSIFICATION OF ARTHRITIS

Chronic Polyarthritis Disease

* Osteoarthritis
* Internal derangement
  * Torn meniscus
  * Osteochondritis
  * Loose body
* Synovitis of unknown cause
* Rheumatoid arthritis
* Traumatic synovitis
* Spondyloarthropathy
* Chondrocalcinosis
* Chronic infection
* Tumour
* Pigmented villonodular synovitis

Chronic Polyarthritis Disease

* Osteoarthritis
* Rheumatoid arthritis
* Systemic lupus erythematosus
* Reiter's syndrome

* Ankylosing spondylitis
* Psoriatic arthritis

GOUT

* Torntmasi's sign :

  Gout—Alopecia on the postero-external aspect of legs (exclusively found in males).
* Acute gouty arthritis is definitely established by identification of monosodium urate monohydrate crystals.

Minor Criteria :

1. More than one attack of acute arthritis.
2. Maximal inflammation developed within 1 day.
3. Attack of monoarticular arthritis.
4. Joints redness observed.
5. First MTP joint painful or sudden.
6. Unilateral attack involving first MTP joint.
7. Unilateral attack involving tarsal joint.
8. Suspected tophus.
9. Hyperuricemia.
10. Asymmetric swelling within a joint (X-ray).
11. Subcortical cysts without erosions (X-ray).
12. Negative culture of joint fluid for microorganism during attack of joint inflammation.

Major Criteria :

1. The presence of characteristic urate crystals in joint fluid.
2. A tophus proved to contain urate crystals by chemical means or polarized light microscopy.

* Acute gouty arthritis require - 1 major and 6 minor criteria for diagnosis.

IMPORTANT POINTS

* Polyarthropathy is seen in sarcoidosis.
* Gout disease will show punched-out appearance of hands on X-ray.

* Juvenile rheumatoid arthritis is called Still's disease.
* Charot's joint is a painless condition.
* Rheumatic nodules are not always associated with active rheumatic carditis.
* Clutton's joint is seen in congenital syphilis.
* Dryness of mouth and eyes with rheumatoid arthritis is seen in Sjogren's syndrome.
* In Duchenne myopathy females carry the disease.
* Cutaneous major manifestation of rheumatic fever is erythema marginatum.
* Most common cause of hypertrophic osteoarthropathy is carcinoma lung.
* Salicylates should be tried first in rheumatoid arthritis.
* Deforming and persistent arthritis is not specific for brucellosis.
* Parrots pseudoparalysis, Clutton's joint and Neuropathic joint are seen in syphilitic arthritis.
* **Pathergy test** is pathognomic of Behcet's syndrome.
* The serological markers for Sjogren's syndrome are Anti ss-A and SS-B.
* The onion skin lesions in the spleen are seen in SLE.
* Most common tendon to rupture is achilles.
* Common toxic manifestation of gold therapy (chrysotherapy) is dermatitis.
* The **commonest** joint involved in Still's disease is Apophyseal joint of cervical spine (notably C2 C3)
* Keratoconjunctivitis sicca, a component of Sjogren's syndrome is diagnosed by Schirmer's test.
* The most common renal lesion of rheumatoid arthritis is amyloidosis.
* The most frequent primary myopathy in adults is dymyositis.
* The most frequent adverse effect of allopurinol in gouty arthritis treatment is precipitation of ac. gouty arthritis.
* The white cell count is normal or slightly elevated in rheumatoid arthritis, but leukopenia may occur, especially in the presence of splenomegaly in Felty's syndrome.
* Mononeuritis multiplex is a characteristic finding of Polyarteritis nodosa.

D/D. OF ARTHRITIS IN CHILDHOOD

Condition	Mono-articular	Polyarticular
a) **Trauma**	+	
b) **Infection**		
- Septic arthritis.		
(Staph. aureus, H. influenzae,	+	+
Meningococcus, Gonococcus	±	
Mycobacteria)	+	
- Virus related		
rubella, hepatitis	+	+
- Osteomyelitis		
c) **Childhood malignant disease**		
- Leukaemia, neuroblastoma	+	+
d) **Haematologic disorder**		
- Haemophilia	+	+
- Sickle cell disease	+	+
e) **Rheumatic disease**		
- Juvenile rheumatoid arthritis	+	+
- Spondyloarthropathies		
Juvenile ankylosing spondylitis	+	+
Arthritis with inflammatory bowel disease	+	+
Reactive arthritis		
Reiter's syndrome	+	+
Postinfectious	+	+
(Salmonella, Shigella, Yerisinea)	+	+
Psoriatic arthritis		
SLE	+	
Dermatomyositis	+	
Scleroderma	+	
Mixed connective tissue disease		
Vasculitic syndromes		
- Henoch-Schonlein purpura	+	

(Contd...)

D/D. OF ARTHRITIS IN CHILDHOOD (Contd....)

	Condition	Mono-articular	Polyarticular
-	Kawasaki disease	+	
-	PAN	+	
-	Behcet's syndrome	+	
-	Rheumatic fever	+	
f.	**Miscellaneous conditions**		
	- Transient synovitis	+	
	- Orthopaedic condittions		
	Slipped capital upper femoral epiphysis	+	
	Perthe's disease	+	
	Osteoid osteoma	+	
	Osteochondritis syndromes	+	
	Chondromalacia patellae	+	
	- Serum sickness		+
	- Non-inflammatory conditions		+
	Limb pains (growing pains)	+	+
	Psychogenic	±	+
	Lyme arthritis	+	±

Normal range of motion of various joints in children

Joint	*Flexion*	*Extension*	*Internal rotation*	*External rotation*	*Abduction*	*Adduction*
Hip	120°	30°	35°	45°	45 to 50°	20-30°
Knee	135°	2-10°	10°	10°	0	0
Ankle	50°	20°	—	—	—	—
Subtalar midtarsal	—	—	5° inversion	5° eversion	10° fore foot	20°
First MTP	45°	70-90°	—	—	—	—
Wrist	80°	70°	—	—	20° radial deviation	30° ulnar deviation
Elbow	135°	0-5°	90° supination	90° pronation	—	—
Shoulder	90°	45°	55°	40-45°	180°	45°
MCPs	90°	30-35°	—	—	—	—
Thumb	70° palmar	0	—	—	20°	0
Neck	45°	50°	80° right	80° left	40° lateral bend	40° lateral bend

Juvenile Rheumatoid Arthritis (JRA)

1. **Diagnostic criteria for JRA**

   a) Arthritis in one or more joints for at least 6 weeks.

   b) Onset < 16 years.

   c) Exclusion of other rheumatic diseases

2. **Classification of Juvenile rheumatoid arthritis**

   Systemic — fever, rash, hepatosplenomegaly, lymphadenopathy, serositis, leucocytosis, anaemia.

   Polyarticular — five or more joints.

   Pauciarticular — four or fewer joints.

Note : This classification is based on clinical presentation within first 6 months after onset of disease.

Spondyloarthropathies

— No accepted diagnostic criteria in children.

— Prototype-Juvenile ankylosing spondylitis.

— May be associated with inflammatory bowel disease or psoriasis or may follow gastrointestinal or genitourinary infection.

C/F includes :

1. Age—Late childhood, earely adolescence.
2. M : F > 6 : 1.
3. F/H of related disease.
4. **Peripheral arthritis**—Pauciarticular, asymmetric, lower extremities most commonly involved.
5. **Axial arthritis**—Often occurs late, sacroiliac or lumbosacral spinal symptoms only in 20% at onset.
6. **Enthesitis** — Tenderness at sites of insertion of tendons and ligaments to bone, e.g. heel pain at Achilles tendon insertion.
7. Absence of ANA and RF.
8. HLA-B27 in 90%

Note : Early stages of JAS may be indistinguishable from pauciarticular JRA.

Dermatomyositis

Diagnostic criteria

1. Symmetric, progressive proximal muscle weakness.
2. Classic dermatomyositis rash.
   — Swelling and heliotrope hue of upper eyelids.
   — Erythematous or violaceous eruption over extensor surfaces, particularly interphalangeal joints, elbows, and knees.
3. Serum muscle enzyme elevation- CPK, aldolase, AST (SGOT), and LDH.
4. EMG evidence of myositis.
5. Muscle biopsy findings typical of dermatomyositis.

Mixed Connective Tissue Diseases (MCTD)

Comprises a syndrome of a combination of F/O:

1. SLE
2. Scleroderma (high incidence of Raynaud's phenomenon, abnormal oesophageal motility, sclerodactyly, and lung disease).
3. Dermatomyositis or Polymyositis
4. Prominent arthritis.

ANA profile

a) High titer antibody to RNP
b) Absence of other ANAs.

Systemic Lupus Erythematosus

Criteria for diagnosing a case of SLE

Malar rash

Discoid rash

Photosensitivity

Oral or nasopharyngeal ulcers

Arthritis-involving 2 or more peripheral joints.

Serositis

a) Pleuritis or
b) Pericarditis

Renal disorder

a) Persistent proteinuria (> 0.5 gm/day or > 3+) or

b) Cellular casts

Neurologic disorder

a) Seizure or

b) Psychosis in absence of offending drugs or metabolic abnormalities.

Haematologic disorder

a) Haemolytic anaemia

b) Leukopenia — < 4.0 x 10^9/L (< 4,000/cmm)

c) Lymphopenia — 1.5 x 10^9/L (< 1,500/cmm)

d) Thrombocytopenia < 100 x 10^9/L (<100,000/cmm) in absence of offending drugs.

Immunologic disorders

a. Positive LE cell preparation or

b. Anti-n DNA antibody or (n-nuclear)

c. Anti-Sm antibody serologic test for syphilis.

ANA—in absence of drugs associated with "drug-induced lupus syndrome."

Diagnosis—Requires 4 or more of these 11 criterias serially or simultaneously.

Additional features to be considered in diagnosed of SLE :

— Raynaud's phenomenon

— Alopecia.

— Constitutional symptoms—fever, lymphadenopathy, hepato-splenomegaly.

Autoantibodies in SLE

Antibody	*Prevalence in SLE*	*Fluorescent staining patterns*	*Other Disease Associations*	*Clinical Associations*
Anti-n DNA (anti-double stranded DNA)	4-60%	Peripheral or rim	Specific for SLE	Renal disease Hypocomplementemia. Worse prognosis.

(Contd....)

Autoantibodies in SLE (Contd...)

Antibody	*Prevalence in SLE*	*Fluorescent staining patterns*	*Other Disease Associations*	*Clinical Associations*
Anti-Sm	25-30%	Speckled	Specific for SLE	Better prognosis if anti-n DNA absent.
Anti-n-RNP	30-35%	Speckled	Not specific for SLE, 100% in MCTD	Arthritis Raynaud's phenomenon, Sclerodactyly serositis, myositis, – prevalence of renal disease Better prognosis
Anti-histones	60%	Homogenous lupus, Sjogren's syndrome,	Drug-induced Subacute ANA negative lupus. Neonatal lupus, SLE with homozygous C2 and C4 deficiency.	Photosensitivity Cutaneous lupus.
Anti-La (anti-SSB)	10-15%	Sjogren's syndrome, Neonatal lupus	Almost always associated with anti-Ro.	

Henoch-Schonlein Purpura or Anaphylactoid Purpura

C/F includes :

1. **Skin lesions (100%)**
   a) Nonthrombocytópenic purpura, particularly over buttocks and lower limbs : necessary for diagnosis.
   b) Angioedema
2. **Arthritis-arthralgia (in - 2/3rd of cases)**
   a) Involves large joints, especially knees and ankles
   b) Frequently periarticular swelling present.
   c) Transient
3. **GIT involvement (in - 2/3rd of cases)**
   a) Colicky abdominal pain may precede arthritis and purpura.
   b) Intussusception and significant haemorrhage (in <5% of cases).

4. **Renal involvement (in - 40% cases)**
   a. Nephritis with haematuria or proteinuria.
   b. Progressive renal failure (in < 5% of cases).
5. **CNS involvement**
6. **Acute scrotal swelling**

Management

1. Supportive + Symptomatic T/t
2. Steroids (Prednisolone) may be indicated for :
   a) Severe GIT involvement
   b) Severe CNS involvement
   c) Severe renal involvement
   d) Severely painful soft tissue swelling
   e) Scrotal or testicular involvement

Important points

— **Commonest** cause of Acute osteomyelitis in a case of sickle cell anemia is Salmonella.

— **Commonest** organism of Acute osteomyelitis organism in children below 3 years is Staphylococcus.

— **Commonest** site of Acute Osteomyelitis in infant is Hip Joint.

— **Commonest** site of Acute Osteomyelitis in children is Femur & Tibia.

— Pain is the most common symptom of musculoskeletal disorders.

— **Achondroplasia** is the most common form of dwarfism. It is autosomal dominant.

— **Lyme arthritis** is a tick borne arthritis caused by a spirochete Borrelia burghdorferi.

— **Most common** site of chondroblastoma is epiphysis.

— **Triradiate pelvis** is seen in Rickets.

— **Calcification of menisci** is seen in Pseudo gout.

— **Pseudofracture** is seen in osteomalacia.

— Most common cause of loose bodies in joints is osteochondritis dissecans.

— Treatment of fracture head of radius in young is immobilization in cast and in elderly is excision of head.

— Fracture of surgical neck of humerus causes injury to axillary nerve leading to loss of roundness of shoulder.

— **Rocker bottom foot** is due to congenital vertical talus.

— **Burton's disease** consists of scurvy and rickets.

— Chemical synovectomy is done by osmic acid.

— Mandible is commonly fractured through cannine fossa.

— In Volkman's ischaemic contracture, flexors of forearm is mainly involved and treatment should be started immediately after suspicion.

— Increased density of bone may be seen in hypervitaminosis.

Lobster hand

— A rare variety of phocomelia, in which hand has only thumb & one finger.

— No treatment is indicated.

Sprengel's shoulder

— Whole shoulder girdle, particularly scapula is higher on affected side, than on the opposite side.

— No treatment is indicated.

Nail-Patella syndrome

— A familial disorder in which nails are hypoplastic or absent & patella is small.

— It is also called **Osteo-onychondysplasia.**

Marble bones (Osteopetrosis, **Albers-Schonberg disease**)

— Familial disease.

— Bone appears dense & structureless.

— Medullary canal absent

Brittle bones (Osteogenesis-Imperfecta)

— Bones are fragile

— Sclera of eye is **blue**

— **Multiple Fractures** are seen.

— Long bones are osteoporotic.

— Bones are **histologically normal.**

Multiple Exostosis (Diaphyseal Aclasis)

— Familial disorder.
— More common in males.
— Due to failure of bone remodelling at the metaphysis.
— Usually develops in **metaphysis** of long bones.
— Exostosis **stop growing** at the completion of skeletal growth.
— 5% of Exostosis undergo malignant changes.
— Surgery (removed en bloc) is done for painful exostosis.

Cleido Cranial Dysostosis (Anosteoplasia)

— Faulty development of membranous bones, mainly of clavicle & skull.
— In some of the cases, clavicles are completely absent so that patient can bring his shoulder in front of chest.

Congenital Torticollis

— Infarction of central portion of sternomastoid muscle at birth.
— Infarcted muscle is replaced by fibrous tissue which contracts.
— As a result face is directed away from the side of lesion.

Commonest Tendon which are liable to rupture

— Supra spinatus
— Biceps brachii
— Rectus femoris
— Tendo achillis

de Quervain's disease

— Stenosing teno vaginitis of common sheath of **Abductor Pollicis Longus & Extensor Pollicis Brevis** tendons of wrist.

Trigger Finger

— Stenosis teno vainitis of flexor tendons of fingers & thumb in the palm.

Ganglia

— Localised, tense, painless, cystic swelling.
— Contain gelatinous fluid.
— Thought to be caused by leakage of synovial fluid through capsule of a joint or tendon sheath.

— Most commonly seen on the dorsum of wrist & foot.

— T/t is excision

Baker's cyst

— Mostly bilateral.

— Centrally placed at post. aspect of popliteal fossa.

— Chronic. cystic swelling, painful, nonpulsatile.

— More prominent on extension of knee.

— Scan, arthrogram will confirm diagnosis in which features of R.A. will be present.

— **T/t**—> resolve spontaneously, if R.A is controlled.

—> it causing disability, aspirated.

Neuropathic joint

— Tertiary syphilis

— Syringomyelia

— Peripheral neuritis (Diabetes)

— Congenital —> Rare cause.

Keller's operation

— For hallux valgus.

— It is excision arthroplasty of base of proximal phalanx.

Mayo's operation

— Done for hallux valgus.

— Excision arthroplasty of head of first metatarsal.

Morton's metatarsalgia

— Most commonly affects fourth toe.

— Main cause is inter-metatarsal bursitis comprising the intermetatarsal nerve.

— **T/t** —> exicison of bursa and affected nerve.

Subungal exostosis

— Most common on the great toe.

— It is painful.

— T/t —> removal of nail & exostosis.

Acute osteomyelitis

— Common in children.

— Commonest organism involved is **staphylococcus aureus.**

— Blood borne infection (Haematogenous).

— Lowered general resistance & local trauma is predisposing factor.

— Disease always begins in **metaphysis.**

— Infective proceses passes through Haversian canals & causing thrombosis of vessels in bone.

— In the first 24 or 48 hrs after infection, exudate forms deep to periosteum.

— Bone infarct in osteomyelitis is known as **sequestrum** (dead piece of bone).

— Involucrum is new piece of bone which surrounds the sequestrum.

— Involucrum has numerous holes which is known as cloaca.

— **Pain** is the presenting symptom.

— Toxicity depends upon virulence of organism.

— Localized tenderness is very important physical signs.

— Movement of joint is permitted to some extend while it is not permitted at all in case of acute suppurative arthritis.

— Blood culture is undertaken before antibiotic treatment started (very important).

— ESR & white cell count is raised but is non-specific.

— No radiological abnormality is seen in first few days of infection.

— New bone can be seen 2-3 weeks after onset of disease.

— If patient is diagnosed within 48 hours antibiotic is the choice of treatment according to sensitivity of organism.

— If patient is diagnosed **after 48 hours,** then surgical evacuation of pus is treatment of choice since pus is usually present by this time.

Chronic osteomyelitis

— Acute haematogenous osteomyelitis pass into chronic osteomyelitis if early treatment is not given or when given it is inadequate.

— Chronic osteomyelitis is in two forms :

(a) When large volume of bone is involved. This is uncommon because of vigorous treatment with antibiotics of early infection.

(b) **Brodie's abscess.** It is **commonest** form of chronic osteomyelitis.

* Composed of pus or gelly like granulation tissue surrounded by sclerotic bone.

* Abscess in case of Brodie's abscess never close by collapse of walls as in soft tissue.

— Osteomyelitis of spine is most commonly caused by **Tuberculosis.**

— Treatment consists of :

(a) Immobilisation of limb

(b) Antibiotics

(c) Surgical removal of dead bone & elimination of dead space.

* Sclerotic bone is removed en bloc.

* Amputation done, if infection is frequent or much prolonged.

Tuberculous Arthritis

— **Haematogenous** in origin.

— In most of the cases, primary focus is related either to the GIT or to the lungs.

— Disease starts either in the **synovial membrane** or in intra-articular bone.

— Commonest site in adult is **spine.**

— Tuberculosis of spine is called **Pott's disease.**

— **Vertebral bodies** are involved first.

— **Tubercles** develop in synovial membrane which is inflammed and infected effusion collects in synovial cavity.

— Articular cartilage is destroyed & adjacent bone is involved.

— Commonest vertebrae involved in **Pott's disease** are T_{9-12}

— Combination of pus formation and spinal angulation (Kyphus) may damage the spinal cord, which may result in **Pott's paraplegia.**

— Tuberculous arthritis in advanced cases causes **fibrous ankylosis.**
— **Pain** is first symptom which is worsened on exertion or at night.
— As the disease progresses, joint becomes stiff because movement is painful. Muscle spasm & bone destruction also present.
— **Kyphus** formation occurs late in Pott's disease.
— If joint is superficial, synovial thickening & effusion is evident.
— Skin overlying joint is not red and is only slightly warmed even if abscess formation has occurred. This feature is very much characteristic of tuberculous inflammation and abscess formation. Such abscesses are called **Cold Abscess.**
— Early Radiological signs are not very much convincing.
— As the disease progresses, there may be narrowing of Joint spaces & bony destructions are visible radiologically.
— Earliest signs in X-ray in Pott's disease is narrowing of disc space.
— Chest X-ray is very important in such cases.
— Bacteriology is confirmatory.
— Antikoch's drugs are treatment of choice.
— But if abscess forms, it requires evacuation, but joint will never regain its normal function.
— Surgery is not required at the synovial stage of disease, since on this stage disease is cured by antibiotics.
— When synovial membrane is very much inflammed & thickened, synovectomy is T/t of choice.
— In spine, some forms of arthrodesis is nearly always required.
— **Melon seed bodies** arise from tuberculous synovitis at the wrist.

MAJOR GROUPS OF THE RHEUMATIC DISEASES

Group	*Diseases*
* Inflammatory arthritis of unknown aetiology	Rheumatoid arthritis Seronegative arthropathies; ankylosing spondylitis, Reiter's syndrome, psoriatic arthritis, enteropathic arthritis

(Contd....)

MAJOR GROUPS OF THE RHEUMATIC DISEASES (Contd.)

	Group	*Diseases*
*	Connective tissue disease	Systemic lupus erythematosus Scleroderma, progressive systemic sclerosis. The arteritides; polyarteritis nodosa, other forms of arteritis. Dermatomyositis and polymyositis, Sjogren's syndrome
*	Crystal deposition disease	Gout Pseudogout Others
*	Degenerative joint disease	Primary Secondary
*	Arthritis associated with infection	Septic arthritis Non-septic arthritis occurring in association with recognised infections; *bacterial*, viral e.g rubella, hepatitis, mumps; *others*, e.g., fungal, protozoal etc. Post-infective arthritis; rheumatic fever, post-salmonella and shigella.
*	Arthritis associated with systemic disease	Cardiovascular; bacterial endocarditis. Endocrine; acromegaly, thyroid and parathyroid disease, diabetes. *Gastroenterological* : Inflammatory bowel disease, Whipple's disease. *Haemopoietic;* Haemophilia, haemoglobinopathies, leukaemia, myeloma. *Heritable developmental and storage diseases:* Marfan's syndrome, hypermobility syndrome. *Immunological* : Hypogammaglobulinaemia, serum sickness.

(Contd....)

MAJOR GROUPS OF THE RHEUMATIC DISEASES (Contd.)

Group	*Diseases*
	Metabolic; Haemochromatosis, hyperlipoproteinaemia
	Metabolic bone disease : Osteoporosis, osteomalacia
	Neurological : Neuropathic arthropathy
	Renal : Chronic renal failure, chronic dialysis
	Respiratory : Hypertrophic pulmonary osteoarthropathy
	Miscellaneous : Sarcoidosis, amyloidosis
* Non-articular rheumatism	Tenosynovitis, bursitis, fibrositis and localised pain Enthesopathies; tennis elbow
	Entrapment neuropathies; carpal tunnel syndrome
	Postural and post-traumatic syndromes
	Localised pain syndrome: shoulder pain, foot pain

Commonest Rheumatic Disease

Non-articular rheumatic syndromes-soft tissue rheumatism.

Degenerative joint disease including spondylosis and disc disease.

Rheumatoid arthritis

Gout

Systemic lupus erythematosus

Rheumatic diseases requiring early recognition and treatment

Septic arthritis

Juvenile chronic polyarthritis

Polymyalgia rheumatica with giant cell arteritis.

Rheumatoid arthritis

HLA ANTIGENS AND ARTHRITIS

Disease	*HLA antigens*	*% Patients*	*% Controls*
Ankylosing spondylitis	B27	90-95	6-10
Reiter's syndrome	B27	75-90	6-10
Psoriatic arthritis			
with peripheral arthritis	B27	10-20	6-10
with spondylitis	B27	50-60	6-10
Inflammatory bowel disease			
peripheral arthritis	B27	6-8	6-10
spondylitis	B27	50-60	6-10
Reactive arthritis			
Salmonella, Yerisinia	B27	70-90	6-10
Rheumatoid arthritis	Dw4	35-55	10-20
	DR4	50-80	20-40

CLINICAL SIGNIFICANCE OF HLA

Even in the case of the strongest HLA association—that of HLA-B27 in ankylosing spondylitis—the presence of the antigen cannot be used as a diagnostic test. Since B27 is present in 6-10% of the control population and ankylosing spondylitis occurs in not more than 20% of individuals with the antigen, the majority of those with HLA-B27 will be free of disease. Thus the 'false positivity' of HLA-B27 renders it unsatisfactory as a diagnostic investigation.

Clinical situations in which HLA-B27 may be useful include :

1. The patient with low back pain who lacks HLA-B27 is unlikely to have ankylosing spondylitis in the absence of psoriasis or inflammatory bowel disease.
2. The young patient with suggestive symptoms but inconclusive X-rays who is HLA-B27 positive should be followed-up carefully.
3. The child, particularly a teenage boy, with lower limb pauciarticular arthritis who is HLA-B27 positive is more likely to follow the course of ankylosing spondylitis than that of typical juvenile arthritis.

BACTERIA LIKELY TO CAUSE SEPTIC ARTHRITIS

Patient	*Organism*
Child	
Neonate	S. aureus E. coli
Age 1 month - 2 years	H. influenzae S. aureus
Age 2 years +	S. aureus Various enteric organisms H. influenzae
Adult	
Healthy	N. gonococcus
RA	S. aureus
Alcohol and drug abuse	S. aureus S. pneumoniae Various enteric organism Pseudomonas, Serratia

NORMAL SYNOVIAL FLUID

Synovial fluid	*Average Value*	*Range*
Volume (in knee) (ml)	2	0.1-4.0
Total protein (g/l)	20	10-30
Leucocytes/mm^3	< 200	30-200
Lymphocytes (%)	50	20-80
Mononuclear (%)	15	2-40
Polymorphs (%)	< 25	10-60
Glucose		
Uric acid	Approximately the same as plasma	
	Electrolytes	

— Lysosomal enzymes present in very low concentration and correlate roughly with the cell count cells; total leucocyte count usually less than 150/mm^3, predominantly lymphocytes with some monocytes and polymorphonuclear cells, also occasional synovial lining cells.

Functions

Lubricates the joint and supplies nutriment to avascular articular cartilage.

SAMPLE ANALYSIS OF SYNOVIAL FLUID

Description	*Normal*	*Non-inflammatory*	*Inflammatory*	*Septic*
Colour	Colourless straw	Straw-yellow	Off-white yellow	Variable
Clarity	Clear	Clear	Translucent opaque	Opaque turbid
Viscosity	High	High	Low	Variable
WBC				
No. mm^3	<200	200-2000	3000-75000	> 50000
% PMNL	< 25	< 25	> 50	> 90

CLASSIFICATION OF SYNOVIAL EFFUSIONS BY TOTAL LEUKOCYTE COUNT

	Normal	*Non-inflammatory* (Group-I)	*Inflammatory* (Group-II)	*Septic* (Group-III)
WBC/mm^3	< 200	200-2000	2,000-75,000	> 100,000

DIFFERENTIAL DIAGNOSIS OF THE FOUR GROUPS OF SYNOVIAL FLUID

Non inflammatory (Group-I)	*Inflammatory (Group-II)*	*Septic (Group-III)*	*Haemorrhagic (Group-IV)*
Degenerative joint disease	Rheumatoid arthritis	Bacterial infections	Trauma
Chronic gout	Seronegative Spondyloarthropathies		Hemophilia
Anticoagulation			
Chronic pseudogout	Acute gout		Tumors
SLE	Acute pseudogout		
Rheumatic fever	SLE		
Progressive systemic sclerosis	Progressive systemic sclerosis		
Trauma	Rheumatic fever		
Osteochondritis dissecans	Partially treated bacterial infection		
Polymyositis	Fungal infections		
	Viral infections		
	Polymyositis		

IMPORTANT TEXT OF SPECIFIC DISORDERS
RHEUMATOID ARTHRITIS

A common and widespread chronic polyarthritis characterized by bilateral symmetrical joint involvement erosions on X-ray, positive tests for rheumatoid factor, and pathologically a chronic proliferative synovitis with villous hypertrophy, infiltration of lymphocytes and plasma cells, and lymphoid nodules.

Incidence

Three percent of females; 1 per cent of males; world-wide.

Onset age 16-70, *commonest* 20-55.

Joints affected

Initially polyarticular in 75 per cent affecting small joints of hands or feet (60 percent), large joints (30 percent) or both (15 percent). Twenty-five per cent monoarticular affecting *knee most commonly* (50 percent), sometimes shoulder, wrist or hip (40 per cent) ankle or elbow (10 percent), small joints rarely.

Ultimately affects hands (PIP joints in 85 percent, MCP in 70 percent, and wrist 80 percent) predominantly. Commonly knees (80 percent). Often ankles (70 percent), shoulders (60 percent), MTP joints and toes (60 percent), elbows (50 percent), cervical spine (50 percent) and hips (40 percent).

Rarely crico-arytenoid joints.

Usually bilateral and symmetrical eventually.

Symptoms

Insidious onset of joint pains and stiffness. Fifteen percent starts with an acute arthritis. Generalized morning stiffness usual, lasting upto 6 hours.

Often accompanied by general ill health, fatigue and weight loss, which may precede joint symptoms by a few months.

Signs

1. Affected joints are usually swollen and tender with limitation of movement. Swelling due to effusion (40 percent) or synovial thickening in early cases and to bony overgrowth in late 'burnt-out' cases.

2. Signs of acute inflammation such as warmth (20 percent) and erythema (10 percent), particularly in early stages and with exacerbations.
3. Muscle wasting around affected joints.

Special features of individual joints

Hands : Ulnar deviation at MCP joints develops between 1 and 5 years after onset. Less common are boutonniere (flexion at PIP joint) and swan-neck (hyperextension at PIP joint) deformities of fingers. Rarely there is arthritis mutilians with main-en-lorgnette ***(opera-glass hand)*** due to bone destruction and soft-tissue excess.

Wrist : Prominent tender ulnar styloid process, with pain on pronation/ supination.

Knees : Baker's cyst (Cystic swelling in popliteal fossa) common. Flexion or valgus deformity and unstability may occur later.

Feet : Tender prominent metatarsal heads with secondary corns; lateral deviation and overriding of toes with pressure sores.

(Cervical spine : Atlanto-axial subluxation present in 30 percent of hospital cases causing pain and very rarely spinal cord compression or vertebral artery occlusion. Crico-arytenoid joint involvement causes hoarseness, stridor, dyspnoea, dysphagia and recurrent bronchitis; sedative dangerous; tracheostomy occasionally required.

Course and prognosis

For the patient with early R.A, there are no accurate guides as to the course the disease will follow :

Although, there is marked individual variation, the following features are associated with a worse prognosis :

— insidious onset
— persistent disease activity
— young age at onset
— seropositivity
— early erosive changes
— marked systemic features.

Non-articular manisfestations

Periarticular soft tissues

1. Nodules (20 percent) usually below elbows but almost anywhere else.
2. Tenosynovitis around hands or wrists (65 percent) causing pain, swelling tenderness, trigger finger, dysfunction and flexion deformity.
3. Bursitis (common), particularly olecranon, causes swelling and discomfort.
4. Synovial cysts appear around any joint but particularly posterior to the knee (Baker's cyst). Raised pressure in knees with large effusions forces fluid into the cyst and may also cause joint rupture with calf pain, ankle oedema and positive Hoffman's sign resembling deep-vein thrombosis.
5. Muscle wasting.
6. Ligamentous laxity leads to hypermobility and deformities, particularly important in causing ulnar deviation and atlanto-axial subluxation.

Skin.

1. Tight, wasted skin common over fingertips (not unlike scleroderma).
2. Leg ulcers (rarely), due to trauma (especially in patients on steroids). hypostasis or associated with vasculitis and Felty's syndrome.

Eyes

1. Scleritis, episcleritis and scleromalacia performs - rare, but may lead to loss of vision.
2. Sjogren's syndrome (15 percent): dry eyes and mouth: confirm by Schirmer's test or Rose Bengal staining; associated with high incidence of allergic reaction, hyperglobulinaemia, auto-antibodies, etc.

Heart

1. Granulomatous lesions in myocardium and valves (rarely cause heart failure), valve lesions (particularly aortic incompetence) and mural thrombi with embolism.
2. Pericarditis : Rub audible at some time in about 10 percent; rarely constrictive.

Vasculitis

Skin lesions around finger nails in 5 percent; rarely gangrene of fingers or toes.

Neuropathy

1. Compression: Carpal tunnel syndrome (50 percent) shortly before or after onset of arthritis.
2. Symmetrical sensorimotor (5 percent) usually affecting legs.
3. Digital : Patchy sensory loss over tips of fingers and toes.
4. Autonomic (rare).
5. Mononeuritis multiplex in association with rheumatoid vasculitis.

Lymphadenopathy (30 percent) and splenomegaly (rare).

Lung involvement

1. Fibrosing alveolitis (rare).
2. Pleural effusion : 8 percent of men; may be the presenting feature of rheumatoid arthritis. Fluid may have low glucose; positive latex test or 'rheumatoid' cells suggestive but not diagnostic.
3. Nodules in lungs or pleura.
4. Caplan's syndrome (multiple pulmonary nodules on chest X-ray in coal-mine workers, iron-foundry workers, etc.).
5. Increased incidence of small airway obstruction in smokers.
6. Rarely acute pneumonitis.

Anaemia

Common and proportional to disease activity. Multiple causation includes failure of marrow iron utilization (anaemia of infection) and aspirin.

Felty's syndrome : Splenomegaly and leucopenia; infections commons.

Infections

Joints commonest site; Staphylococcus aureus commonest organism; may be silent, and not always accompanied by fever or leucocytosis.

Oedema

1. Localized chronic oedema of one hand or forearm (rare).
2. Ankle oedema (10 percent) with active disease.

Osteoporosis and fractures

Aggravated by steroid therapy; important cause of sudden worsening of pain in one joint.

Amyloidosis

Presents as proteinuria; may progress to renal failure.

Diagnosis by rectal, fat or renal biopsy.

Radiography

Early :

1. Periarticular osteoporosis.
2. Erosions : Changes best seen in X-ray of hands and feet.

Late :

1. Loss of joint space
2. Bone destruction
3. Rarely ankylosis

Special sites

Cervical spine : Ask for views in flexion and extension; any increase in the distance between the odontoid process and the anterior arch of the atlas in flexion is abnormal and indicates atlanto-axial subluxation.

Hip : Head of femur appears to 'burrow' into the acetabulum and may progress to protrusion acetabuli. Note also absence of sclerosis (c.f. osteoarthritis).

SOME CONDITIONS AND APPROXIMATE FREQUENCY IN WHICH RHEUMATOID FACTOR IS PRESENT

A. *Rheumatic diseases*

Adult rheumatoid arthritis (80%)

Sjogren's syndrome (90%)

Systemic lupus erythematosus (25%)

Scleroderma (20%)

Mixed connective tissue disease (50%)

Polymyositis (20%)

Juvenile rheumatoid arthritis (10-25%)

B. *Acute viral infections*

Infectious mononucleosis (variable)

Infective hepatitis (25%)

Influenza (variable)

Rubella (variable)

C. *Chronic inflammatory disease*

Tuberculosis (15%)

Syphilis (10%)

Infective endocarditis (40%)

D. *Neoplasma (variable)*

E. *Miscellaneous*

Aged but otherwise normal individuals (15-50%)

Sarcoidosis (25-40%)

Chronic active hepatitis (10-20%)

Chronic persistent hepatitis (10-20%)

Hyperglobulinemic purpura (90%)

After transfusions (variable)

After renal transplantation (variable)

Laboratory

Anaemia and raised ESR common with active disease.

Latex test positive in 80 percent but never anti-DNA antibodies.

Synovial fluid : Often appears purulent (yellow or green and turbid). Low viscosity : WBC up to 100000 x $10^9/1$: mostly neutrophils.

Latex test parallels serum titre and has no diagnostic significance in seronegative cases. Sterile on culture.

Synovial biopsy may show non-specific chronic synovitis or characteristic changes.

Treatment

1. Initiate regular anti-inflammatory therapy to control the symptoms—start with safer drugs like propionic acid derivatives. Try them all if necessary to find the best for each patient.

2. Supplement with simple analgesics on demand, indomethacin at night for morning stiffness, intra-articular steroids for troublesome joints.
3. Suppression of disease activity :
   a) Penicillamine : 250 mg daily. Check WBC, platelets and urine protein at least monthly. Side effects common. For loss of taste or nausea carry on regardless. For rash, vomiting or thrombocytopenia, stop and restart low doses when normal. Proteinuria occurs after 4 months or more; stop if it exceeds 5 g daily or patient becomes nephrotic.
   b) Gold 10, 20, 30, 40 mg i.m. at weekly intervals, then 50 mg weekly up to 1 g then maintenance dose of 50 mg fortnightly, if results good. Check white count and platelets fortnightly, and urine for protein before each injection.
   c) Immunosuppressive drugs : Azathioprine (50 mg b.d.). chlorambucil (5 mg daily). Cyclophosphamide (50- 100 mg daily) reserved for severe or life-threatening disease.
   d) Hydroxychloroquine : 400 mg daily — mild but sometimes useful; 6-monthly eye tests essential.
   e) Salazopyrine : 500 mg twice daily for two weeks then 1 g.b.d. Use enteric coated tablets. Consider combination with penicillamine.
4. Continued supervision and management of complications.

   Carpal tunnel syndrome : Local steroid injection; surgery if this fails.

   Ruptured extensor tendons of hand; repair, debridement and excision of ulnar head.

   Atlanto-axial subluxation : No treatment required; caution if anaesthetic needed; spinal fusion only for definite evidence of cord compression.

   Baker's cyst, calf cyst or joint rupture : Rest, intra-articular steroids and if symptoms are particularly troublesome, synovectomy.

   Felty's syndrome :Avoid steroids; splenectomy may help but benefit often transient; drugs like penicillamine to control the disease.

   Sjogren's syndrome : Hypromellose eye drops.

APPROACH TO DRUG MANAGEMENT IN RHEUMATOID ARTHRITIS

First line

Non-steroidal anti-inflammatory agents

Analgesics

Second line

Hydroxychloroquine

Sulphasalazine

Gold

Penicillamine

Third line

Azathioprine

Methotrexate

Cyclophosphamide

Chlorambucil

Steroids

Intra-articular - useful at any state

Oral - Low dose (5-10 mg) may be used on their own or in combination with disease modifying agents parenteral - used to cover surgery or in life-threatening events such as systemic vasculitis (methyl prednisolone).

— Severity and duration of morning stiffness.

— Soft tissue swelling.

— Degree of 'anaemia of chronic disease'.

— Height of ESR

— Prominent systemic symptoms including malaise, fatigue.

— Recent involvement of new joints.

— Radiological progression of erosions.

SERONEGATIVE ARTHROPATHIES

The term seronegative arthropathies, or seronegative spondyarthritis conventionally includes the following entities :

Ankylosing spondylitis

Reiter's syndrome

Psoriatic arthritis and spondylitis

Enteropathic arthritis and spondylitis

Juvenile chronic arthritis

These disorders, although, clinically distinct and usually easily separated, are unified by two major characteristics: the synovial histology of involved peripheral joints may be indistinguishable from RA but rheumatoid factor is absent.

In addition, there are several features which occur commonly in each entity within the group: sacroiliitis and spondylitis, iritis, mucocutaneous lesions, familial aggregation of single and occasionally multiple seronegative arthropathies, and increased prevalence of HLA-B27. Thus the several clinical features shared by this group of rheumatic diseases appear to be linked by a common genetic thread.

ANKYLOSING SPONDYLITIS

A chronic condition of the spine and sacroiliac joints in which early inflammatory changes causing back pain and stiffness may be followed by progressive restriction of spinal movement associated with radiological calcification of spinal ligaments and sacroiliitis.

Incidence

Affects 1 percent of males and females.

Age at onset 15-30 but rarely earlier or later.

Joints affected

Initially sacroiliacs affected symmetrically and bilaterally with involvement of entire spine thereafter.

Shoulders and hips affected in 40 percent; peripheral joints in 25 percent, knees, commonest (15 percent), also ankles (10 percent). feet (5 percent) and rarely fingers.

Ribs fuse on to vertebrae and transverse processes; sternomanubrial and sternoclavicular joints often affected.

Symptoms

Gradual onset of low backache and/or pain in both buttocks (pseduo-bilateral sciatica). Morning stiffness.

15 percent present with peripheral arthritis.

Signs

1. Restriction of all movements of spine.
2. Chest expansion reduced (<5 cm).
3. Bony Points often tender (heels, sternum, ribs, pelvic brim and ischial tuberosities).
4. Peripheral joints may be swollen and tender.
5. *Schober's test* (Patient standing erect and bending makes a difference of 4 cm or less between 2 points taken in midline from spinous process of L_5 5 cm below and 10 cm above).

Associations

1. Iritis in 25 per cent and other HLA B27-related diseases; juvenile chronic arthritis and Reiter's disease may precede ankylosing spondylitis. Ulcerative colitis and Crohn's disease may precede or follow.
2. Aortic incompetence (1 percent).
   Cardiac conduction defect (8 percent).
3. Plantar fasciitis and other soft-tissue problems.

Rarely :

4. Amyloidosis
5. Atlanto-axial subluxation or fracture of rigid segments of the spine which may be fatal.
6. Apical pulmonary fibrosis resembling pulmonary tuberculosis, associated with recurrent episodes of pneumonitis and pleurisy.
7. Cauda equina syndrome sphincter disturbances, sensory loss in the perineum, and absent ankle jerks.

Radiography

Changes best seen in sacroiliac joints and spine (D10 to L2). Sacroiliititis is essential for diagnosis.

1. *Pelvis :* Sacroiliac joints usually abnormal; sclerosis; blurring or joint outline; later obliteration. Ischial tuberosities roughened and show ***'whiskering'*** with periosteal elevations. Symphasis pubis may be blurred.
2. *Spine : Syndesmophytes;* longitudinal ligamentous calcification eventually producing ***'bamboo'*** spine; lytic lesions appear particularly at the upper anterior corners of vertebral bodies; ***squaring*** of vertebrae.

Laboratory

ESR raised in 80 percent; often mild anaemia, latex test negative. Synovial fluid: inflammatory; WBC up to 20000 x $10^9/1$, mainly neutrophils. Tissue antigen HLA B27 found in 96 percent.

Treatment

1. Exercise and exercises to maintain as full mobility as possible and prevent deformity
2. NSAIDs : Indomethacin particularly useful : 75-100 mg at night for morning stiffness with day-time doses of 25 mg if necessary. Alternative includes flurbiprofen 100 mg at night and piroxicam 20 mg at night. *Never steroids.*
3. Surgery only rarely needed, usually hip replacement. Spinal (wedge lumbar) osteotomy for marked kyphosis.
4. Radiotherapy in conservative dosage helpful but carries risk of leukaemia and best avoided.

DIFFERENTIAL DIAGNOSIS OF ARTHRITIS IN CHILDREN

---

1. Juvenile chronic arthritis of various types (above)
2. Rheumatic fever
3. Henoch-Schonlein disease
4. Acute leukaemia
5. Systemic lupus erythematosus. 15 percent of cases occur in children.
6. Dermatomyositis and scleroderma
7. Psoriatic arthropathy
8. Traumatic arthritis
9. Infections: Septic arthritis, tuberculosis, rubella, mumps etc.
10. Perthes' disease
11. Transient synovitis of the hip
12. Enteropathic synovitis
13. Post-dysenteric Reiter's disease
14. Familial Mediterranean fever

15. Hypogammaglobulinaemia
16. 'Growing pains'-possibly sychogenic and not accompanied by swelling or other objective abnormalities of joints.
17. Erythema nodosum
18. Sickle-cell disease
19. Clutton's joints
20. Plant thorn synovitis

AMERICAN RHEUMATOLOGICAL ASSOCIATION's REVISED CRITERIA FOR CLASSIFICATION OF SLE

Malar rash

Discoid rash

Photosensitivity

Oral/nasal ulcers

Non-deforming arthritis (two or more joints)

Serositis (Pleurisy or pericarditis)

Renal disease

CNS disease

Haematological disease (anaemia, leucopenia, lymphopenia or thrombocytopenia).

Immunological abnormalities (LE cells, anti-ds DNA, anti-Sm, positive VDRL, TPHA).

Antinuclear antibody (by immunofluorescence)

DEGENERATIVE DISEASES
OSTEOARTHRITIS (Osteoarthrosis)

A disorder of cartilage with characteristic histological, clinical and radiological features. The histological changes include flaking of the surface of cartilage (fibrillation), the appearance of vertical fissures and proliferation of chondrocytes which form nests around the fissures. Electron microscopy shows the presence of increased numbers of matrix vesicles which are the site of formation of crystals of hydroxyapatite. There is progressive loss of cartilage and secondary changes in subchondral bone, fibrosis of the capsule and mild inflammatory changes in synovium. Various biochemical changes suggests that the disease may be a metabolic abnormality of cartilage. There is increased water content, loss of proteoglycans, increased levels of potentially destructive enzymes like cathepsin-D and increased excretion of alkaline phosphatase and pyrophosphatase. Some conditions appear to lead to osteoarthritis or to determine its occurrence at a particular site (secondary osteoarthritis).

1. Congenital anatomical aberrations of joints: Hypermobility. Abnormally shaped or positioned surfaces.
2. Structural disorders arising in children: Perthes' disease. Slipped femoral epiphysis.
3. Trauma and mechanical problems: Fractures involving the joint surface. Meniscectomy. Obesity, recurrent dislocation. occupational hazards.
4. Crystal deposition disease: Pyrophosphate arthropathy, Gout.
5. Metabolic abnormalities of cartilage: Ochro-nosis
6. Avascular necrosis
7. Other conditions in which cartilage is destroyed including septic arthritis and recurrent haemarthrosis in haemophilia.

In most cases, the disease is primary, without obvious predisposing cause.

Incidence

Very common - about 20 percent have it.

F : M:: 2 : 1

Peak onset age 50, usually 40-65.

Fifty percent of the population have XR changes - almost universal after age of 55.

About 50 percent of patients with XR changes have symptoms.

FH in 40 percent.

Inheritance probably mulitfactorial.

Joints involved

Knees (75 percent) and hands (60 percent).

Commonest

In the hands, DIP joints and carpometacarpal joints of thumb are commonest with PIP joints (50 percent) less prominent and MCP joints unusual. Feet in 40 percent, usually 1st MTP joint other MTP joints less commonly.

Lumbar (30 percent) and cervical spine (20 percent) often- hips (25 percent) ankles (20 percent) shoulders (15 percent) rarely elbows or wrists. Ten percent monoarticular. Usually one, two, three or four sites. Bilateral in 85 percent - when one is affected first or more severely, it is usually the dominant side.

Symptoms

Pains, worst towards evening and aggravated by particular activities. Eighty percent have morning stiffness (usual 10-30 min. and seldom more than 60 min. - localized to one or two sites) and inactivity stiffness (usually 5 min. and seldom more than 30 min).

Signs

Knee: Bony swelling, effusion in 60 per cent Baker's cryst (409 percent) tenderness painful limitation of movement, crepitus.

DIP joints : Joints often red, warm and exquisitely tender in acute stage (hot Heberden's nodes'). After months or years inflammatory features pass leaving bony swelling and sometime flexion, valgus or varus deformities.

CMC joint : Square hand with bony swelling, tenderness and crepitus of joint.

Others: Bony swelling, tenderness, crepitus, painful limitation of movement.

Course

Chronic additive pattern. Slowly progressive with exacerbations and remissions. Affected joints develop progressive painful restriction of movement, sometimes with deformities (hip-flexion:knee-valgus) or laxity.

Greatest disability in late stages results from involvement of weight-bearing joints.

Associations

No extra-articular features.

XR

1. Loss of joint space.
2. Sclerosis of adjacent bone.
3. Marginal osteophytes.
4. Subarticular cysts.
5. 'Spotty' calcification indicates hydroxyapatite deposition. Seen in the hand 60 percent, usually DIP joints, and knees in 25 percent. 'Linear' calcification (chondrocalcinosis) indicates pyrophosphate deposition.

Laboratory

ESR normal

Latex negative (but 5 percent positive in normal elderly people)

No diagnostic tests

Synovial fluid: clear and viscous

'Non-inflammatory'. Usually about 3000 (up to 15000 x 10^9 cells/I) Typically 80 percent mononuclear (40-100 percent) !look for pyrophosphate crystals under polarized light. Electron microscopy may show cystals of hydroxyapatite.

Treatment

1. Analgesic and anti-inflammatory drugs to relieve pain. Start with propionic acid derivatives. Simple analgesics on demand for patient with mild or intermittent pain.
2. Hip: Total replacement

   Knee: Replacement or osteotomy to relieve pain and correct deformity.

   CMC joint: Trapezectomy or fusion
3. Physical measures: Walking stick. Reduce weight by dieting. Physiotherapy to maintain muscle power and range of movement. Hydrotherapy for painful stiff hips.

Orthopaedic surgery

Indications

1. Severe pain, inadequately controlled by conservative measure.
2. Marked joint instability or functional impairment, preferably accompanied by significant pain.

3. When these occurs in :
   - advanced disease
   - a joint suitable for surgery
   - A patient who wants the operation and has a realistic understanding of what surgery has to offer.

Special considerations

Overweight patients, undergoing surgery on lower limb joints, should loose weight.

Peripheral vascular disease may contraindicate surgery on the knee or foot.

Patients should be willing to undertake the necessary post-operative exercise programme; those with OA of the knee benefit from having strong quadriceps muscle prior to operation.

Surgery on the hip or knee is of limited value if other lower limb joints are too damaged to allow improved functions. In such situations, the operation being considered should, by itself, allow significant symptomatic improvement or it must be planned as one of a series of procedures.

Operations

Basic types of operations involve:

- realignment: osteotomy
- stabilization: arthrodesis
- mobilization: arthroplasty including excision arthroplasty i.e.
- Keller's operation, and replacement.
- arthroplasty, e.g. total hip replacement.

Joints commonly subjected to surgery of established value include:

Hip: Total hip replacement, when performed skillfully on selected patients, is usually a strikingly successful operation.

Knee:

- Osteotomy with or without realignment.
- Replacement arthroplasty; various types, none yet as regularly satisfactory as total hip replacement.

MTP 1: With hallux valgus or hallux rigidus:
- — Removal of exostosis and bunion.
- — Keller's operation, an excision arthroplasty.
- — Arthrodesis of the MTP joint in a slightly extended position

First carpometacarpal joint (base of the thumb)
- — Excision arthroplasty
- — Siliastic interposition arthroplasty

Others : Replacement operations on shoulder or elbow joints are providing successful in some centres.

SECONDARY FORMS OF OA

1. *Inflammatory states* (inflammatory joint disease associated with residual joint damage)
   a) Healed rheumatoid arthritis
   b) Healed Psoriatic arthropathy
   c) Gout
   d) Septic and tuberculous arthritis
   e) Haemophilic arthropathy
2. *Endocrine diseases*
   a) Acromegaly
   b) Diabetes mellitus
   c) Hypothyroidism
3. *Metabolic disorders*
   a) Haemochromatosis
   b) Ochronosis
   c) Mucopolysaccharidosis
   d) Wilson's disease

Congenital Dislocation of the Hip (CDH)

Incidence

The reported incidence of unstable hips is much higher, varying from 8 to 20 per 1,000 live births

Aetiology

Three factors appear to be important in its aetiology:

1. An hereditary predisposition to joint laxity.
2. Female sex on the part of the infant: The condition is 3 to 5 time more common in girls.
3. Breech malposition of the foetus: The incidence of instability of the hip is about 10 times as great as for infants with a vertex presentation.

Clinical features

It is imperative that this condition to be diagnosed in the first few days of life.

Diagnosis at birth

At birth the appearance of the infant is normal, and the hips move fully. Radiologically, the epiphysis of the femoral head does not appear until the first year of life and the acetabulum is largely cartilaginous so that, even if the hip is dislocated rather than dislocateable, there is no obvious radiological abnormality.

The demonstration of Instability of the hip at birth

The demonstration consists of eliciting a click from the hip, and is known as Barlow's or von Rosen's sign.

The hip is flexed to 90° and adducted. Whilst adduction is taking place, gentle pressure is exerted by the examining hand in a proximal direction along the long axis of the femoral shaft. As the femoral head rolls over the posterior lip of the acetabulum it may, if dislocateable (but not if dislocated), slip out of the acetabulum. The sensation which the examing hand receives is composed of a mixture of the feeling of abnormal posterior movement plus a distinct 'clunk' as the femoral head leaves the acetabulum. If the hip is dislocated by this manoeuvre or if it is already dislocated prior to examination, the second half of the physical sign can now be elicited.

The treatment of CDH in the newborn infant

Various splints have been devised by keeping the hip in a position of 90° flexion and abduction (a position in which the femoral head is stable in the acetabulum) for a period of *three months.* All are satisfactory. One such splint is the von Rosen splint.

The diagnosis of CDH in a child of one years' age or more

1. von. Rosen's sign
2. Abnormal skin crease
3. No abduction in 90° flexion
4. Telescoping present
5. Trendelenburg's test positive
6. Lurching gait if unilateral, Wadding gait if bilateral (Rolling-saitor gait)
7. *Radiology* (positive after 1 year)
   * Lateral and upward displacement of epiphyses of femoral head.
   * Break in Shenton's line (i.e. continuous curve produced by inf. margin of superior pubic ramus and medial cortex of femoral neck and shaft).
   * Small capital femoral epiphysis
   * Shallow acetabulum

Treatment between the age of 6 months and 7 years (for unilateral dislocation) or 4 years (for bilateral dislocation).

Weight-bearing at the infant hip begins when the infant crawls at about 6 months. From this age until about 7 years for unilateral dislocation, and about 4 years for bilateral dislocation, it is possible to reduce hip and obtain adequate function.

Treatment aims to replace the femoral head in the acetabulum and to keep it there whilst normal developoment occurs. Reduction is impeded by the fact (1) the soft tissues have by this time developed in such a way as to confirm with the abnormal position of the femur, and (2) the acetabulum has become filled with a mass of fibro-fatty tissue. Maintenance of reduction is difficult because: (1) the acetabulum is abnormally shallow and vertical; (2) the femoral head is smaller than normal and (3) the femoral neck is usually retroverted on the shaft.

Closed 'Manipulation'- The femoral head may reduce spontaneously during a period of traction, or it may be reduced under anaesthesia after a period of traction. Open adductor and sometimes psoas tenotomy is often needed to allows the hip to be fully abducted without forcibly compressing the femoral head.

Maintenance of Reduction - If the hip has been replaced either by closed or open means it must be maintained in the acetabulum from a period of months by some form of splintage. Extreme internal or external rotation should be avoided. After 3 to 6 months a hip spica may be exchanged for a Denis Browne splint if the child is under *2 years of age.*

If reduction has been deferred until the bones of the hip have developed abnormally, surgical reconstruction of the hip may be required in addition to open reduction. The available procedures consist of:

1. *Pelvic Osteotomy* (shelter) which aims to rotate the acetabulum into a more horizontal position to cover the femoral head.
2. *Shelf -Operation* in which the superior hip of the acetabulum is reconstructed (so that it covers the femoral head) by a bone graft or by medial displacement of the acetabulum relatively to the ilium after a pelvic osteotomy just above the hip.
3. *Inter-trochanteric Rotation Osteotomy of the Femur* in which the proximal fragment is rotated, bringing the femoral head squarely into the acetabulum.

Treatment of the older child—Putti suggested that the results of treatment in bilateral dislocations of the hip over the age of 4 years and in unilateral dislocations over the age of 7 years are worse than the results of the disease itself and thus that no treatment is indicated for these children in childhood. A lower age limit applies to bilateral dislocation because: (1) the limp is less noticeable; (2) as a consequence these patients, although they have a slightly abnormal posture and an abnormal gait, tend to live normal lives until they are in 40's when secondary osteoarthrosis may develop; (3) there is a danger that treatment may be more successful in one hip than in the other so that a bilateral dislocation is converted into a unilateral dislocation; and (4) treatment may be stiffen the hip, a tolerable outcome to one hip but a significant disability if it affects both.

CLUB FOOT

Nomenclature— 'Club Foot' is a loose term used to describe a number of different abnormalities in the shape of the foot. If the foot is fixed in a position of plantar-flexion so that it cannot be fully dorsiflexed, the deformity is described as one of 'equinus'. The opposite deformity is described as *'calcaneus'*. If the foot is inverted and adducted at the mid-tarsal joint so that it cannot be fully everted. The opposite deformity is described as *'valgus'*. Almost invariably two or more of the deformities are combined and by far the most common congenital combination is *'equino-varus.* The Latin synonym for club foot is *talipes* and the descriptive nomenclature for a club foot combines this term with the Latin description of the deformity. Thus, the most common variety of congenital club foot is known as *'Talipes Equino-Varus'*.

Aetiology—In the great majority of patients with congenital club foot the aetiology is unknown, and this group should properly be called idiopathic congenital club foot. But because this variety represents the majority of the club foot, it is usually referred to simply as 'congenital club foot'.

Congenital club foot may be paralytic and secondary to myelodysplasia. The deformities in arthogryposis multiplex congenital may also include club foot. The club foot in this disease is gross, and nearly always associated with other deformities, in particular with clubbing of the hand.

Morbid anatomy

1. *Adduction and external rotation of the bones of the forefoot*—The adduction occurs at the mid-tarsal and tarso-matatarsal joints, but also to some extent affects the bones themselves which are curved so as to be concave medially. The adduction may be so gross as to result in medial dislocation of the navicular from the talo-navicular joint. The external rotation is produced by torsion of the shafts of the metatarsal.
2. *Inversion of the os calcis and of the navicular on the talus*—The inverted os calcis and navicular carry the rest of the foot into inversion with them.
3. *Plantar-flexion of all the bones of the foot including the talus*—The talus, although plantar-flexed, is not as plantar-fixed as the other bones so that the head of the talus tends progressively to dislocate from the mid-tarsal joint in a dorsal as well as a lateral direction.
4. There is possibly an early abnormality in the neck of the talus which, it has been suggested, is angulated to that the head of the talus is displaced downwards and medially. Secondary, changes occur in the head of the talus.

5. The os calcis may be small. As a consequence the heel is small.
6. All the ligamentous structures on the medial side of the foot and to some extent in the sole are shortened, but are histologically normal.
7. As a result, the flexors of the foot and toes and the invertors of the foot are short. As growth takes place, hypoplasia commonly persists in spite of effective treatment for the deformity, so that finally the whole of the foot and calf are smaller than normal.
8. The skin shows adaptive shortening on the concave side of the curve.

Clinical features—The condition should be diagnosed at birth. The normal new-born foot has a greater range of dorsiflexion and eversion than the normal adult foot; it can be dorsiflex until the dorsum touches the anterior aspect of the skin. If this is impossible, a minor degree of talipes equino-varus exists. If a club foot is detected, the spine and all other joints should always be examined carefully to exclude myelodysplasia and arthrogryphosis. Since the bones of the foot are at this stage largely cartilagenous, radiography is useless.

Treatment

Conservative Treatment—If the deformity is light, so that the foot can be dorsiflexed to a little beyond the plantigrade position, the mother should be taught to manipulate her child's foot after every feed. Sufficient pressure should be exerted by the mother to blanch her own fingers and this pressure should be maintained for about 2 seconds. The pressure should be released and re-applied over a period of about 5 minutes. Minor deformity can usually be corrected on this regime but the infant should be examined at monthly intervals to ensure that the deformity does infact steadily diminish.

If initially the foot cannot easily be brought beyond the plantigrade position, the maximum correction obtained by manipulation must be maintained and gradually increased by serial splintage. The neonatal foot is too small to be treated satisfactorily in plaster-of-Paris but correction can usually be maintained by strapping. The splint is removed and reapplied with a little more correction (every week). By this method gradual correction of the deformity may be achieved so that, if all goes well, by 3 months the deformity can easily be corrected to beyond the plantigrade position. Splintage is then discontinued and maternal manipulation substituted. If the age of 1 to 2 months the poistion of the foot is not satisfactory, plaster of-Paris is substituted for the aluminium splint. The plaster is changed at **3 weekly** intervals.

On this regime most club foot should have been corrected by the age of about 3 months.

Denis Browne splints may be used throughout the day instead of maternal manipulation until the child walks and thereafter they may be used at night.

Treated by Operation

A minority of club foot cannot be satisfactorily corrected by manipulation and splintage *by the age of 6 weeks.*

The Operation of Medial release and Elongation of the Achilles Tendon for Talipes Equino-Varus

Through a curved incision posterior and distal to the medial malleolus the ligaments on the medial side of the ankle, talonavicular and navicular-cuniform joints are divided. The tendons of tibialis anterior, tibialis posterior, flexor hallucis longus and flexor digitorum longus are divided and elongated by Z-plastry.

Treatment of 'Relapsed Club Foot'- If relapse occurs in a child less than 4 years of age, a soft tissue release as described above is usually sufficient, *but in the children over the age of 6 this procedure is insufficient.* Children presenting with unsatisfactory feet at this age require not only medial release but also resection of bone from the lateral side of the foot.

The lateral rein is shortened by resecting the articular surfaces of calcaneo-cuboid joint and stapling the calcaneum to the cuboid so as to achieve calcaneo-cuboid fusion.

In adolescent children presenting with an unsatisfactory club foot, the foot may be corrected by the resection of laterally based wedges (followed by fusion of the exposed bony surfaces) from the mid-foot to correct forefoot adduction and the os calcis (to correct inversion of the heel).

In the condition presents in adult life, subtalar (triple) fusion with an appropriate resection of bone so as to bring the sole into a plantigrade position is the treatment of choice. Astragalactomy is the alternative if the deformity is severe.

* WORMIAN BONES

Normal (especially lambdoid) suture	Idiopathic osteoarthropathy
Osteogenesis imperfecta	Hallermann-Streiff syndrome
Cleidocranial dysplasia	Aminopterin embryonopathy
Cretinism	Kinky hair or Menkes syndrome
Some trisomies	Cutis aplasia congenitia
Healing rickets	Hadju-Cheny syndrome
Pyknodysostosis	Zeweger syndrome
Hypophosphatasia	Otopalatodigital syndrome
Pachydermoperiostosis	Prader-Willi syndrome
	Progeria

* VERTEBRAL SCALLOPING

Posterior	**Anterior**
Normal-lumbar	Normal-lower thoracic and upper lumbar
Intraspinal tumor, cyst	Neurofibromatosis
Neurofibromatosis	Leukemia, lymphoma
Achondroplasia, other chondrodystrophies	Metastatic disease
Storage diseases	Adjacent intra-abdominal tumors, cysts
Ehler-Danlos syndrome	Dural ectasia
Marfan syndrome	Small canal
Hydromyelia, syringomyelia	Dysplastic vertebra
Uncontrolled communicating hydrocephalus	Destruction
	Erosion

* FLAT VERTEBRAE

Single or multiple but not all vertebral bodies	**All vertebral bodies**
Fracture	Severe osteoporosis-osteomalacia

Eosinophilic granuloma
Histiocytosis-X
Metastatic disease
Congenital variation
Osteogenesis imperfecta
Osteomalacia-osteoporosis
Leukemia-lymphoma
Sickle-cell disease
Severe osteogenesis imperfecta
Other anemias
Leukemia, lymphoma
Spondyloepiphyseal dysplasia
Thanatophoric dwarfism
Metatropic dwarfism
Morquio disease
Achondrogenesis
Kniest syndrome
Dyggva-Melchior-Clausen syndrome

* **CUBOID VERTEBRAE**

Normal achondroplasia
Hypochondroplasia
Other chondrodystrophier
Storage diseases
Short rib-polydactyly syndrome

* **WEDGED VERTEBRAE**

Anterior compression fracture
Scoliosis
Kyphosis
Scheurmann disease
Normal
Hemivertebrae-sagittal
Hemivertebrae-coronal Gibbus
a) Lateral wedging
b) Venous causes
c) Thoracic spine minimal
d) Gibbus
e) Other causes

* **HOOKED OR BREAKED VERTEBRAE**

Normal in infants
Storage diseases
Hypothyroidism
Acute and chronic trauma
Scheuermann disease
Neurogenic or neuromuscular disease with hypotonia
Achondroplasia
Bone dysplasia in neurofibromatosis

* SMALL SQUARED AND FLARED ILIAC WINGS—DECREASED ACETABULAR ANGLE

Type-A Cleidocranial dysostosis

Achondroplasia
Achondrogenesis
Asphyxiating thoracic dystrophy
Elis-van Creveld syndrome
Short rib-polydactyly syndromes
Metatropic dwarfism
Kniest syndrome
Spondyloepiphyseal dysplasia congenita
Punctate epiphyseal dysplastic-rhizomelic form
Thanatophoric dwarfism
Morquio disease
Severe metaphyseal dysostoses
Dyggve-Melchior-Clausen syndrome
Immune deficiency syndromes

Cockayene syndrome
Acrocephalosyndactyly
Aminopterin-induced syndrome
Arthrogryposis
Cornelia de Lange syndrome
Hypophosphatasia
Popliteral pterygium syndrome
Osteo-onchodysplasia
Prune-belly syndrome
Rubinstein-Taybi syndrome
Bladder extrophy
Sacral agenesis
Trisomy-13-18
Metaphyseal dysostosis: mild cases

Type-B Osteogenesis imperfecta

Trisomy-21: Down's syndrome
Mucopolysachharidoses: except Morquio
Mucolipidoses
Other storage diseases

Weissenbacher-Zweymuller syndrome
Larsen syndrome
Congenital dislocating hip
Melnick-Needles syndrome

* IRREGULAR OR FRAGMENTED EPIPHYSES

Hypothyroidism
Normal: distal femur, capitellum
Legg-Perthes' disease
Aseptic necrosis
Rheumatoid arthritis
Hemophilic arthritis

Frost bite of feet and hands
Osteomyelitis of epiphysis
Pigmented villonodular synovitis
Morquio disease
Epiphyseal dysplasia hemimelica:

Multiple epiphyseal dysplasia
Spondyloepiphyseal dysplasia
Aseptic necrosis
- Collagen vascular disease
- Congenital hip treatment
- Gaucher's disease
- After hip surgery
- After septic hip

Trevor disease
Thiemann disease
Tricho-rhino-phalangeal syndrome: femoral head
Dyggve-Melchior-Clausen syndrome
Meyer dysplasia (hips)
Winchester syndrome
Zellweger syndrome

* INDISTINCT AND RINGED EPIPHYSIS

Indistinct Epiphyseal margins
Rickets
Hyperparathyroidism (Sec.)
Hypothyroidism
Primary Hyperparathyroidism
Jansen metaphyseal dysostosis
Mucolipidosis-II
Gangliosidosis

* RINGED EPIPHYSIS

Severe chronic osteoporosis
Healing rickets
Healing hypothyroidism
Osteogenesis imperfecta
Scurvy

* CONE-SHAPED EPIPHYSIS

Normal
Trauma
Infection
Bone infraction
Sickle cell disease
Multiple osteochondromatosis
Metaphyseal dysostosis-dysplasia
Metaphyseal and spondylo-epiphyseal dysplasia
Cleidocranial dysostosis
Acrocephalosyndactyly syndrome
Asphyxiating thoracic dystrophy
Hypophosphatesia

Osteopetrosis
Pseudo-or pseudohyperpara-thyroidism
Vitamin-A intoxication: chronic
Acrodysostosis
Non-specific brachydactyle
Marchesani syndrome
Seckel bird-headed dwarf
Oro-facial-digital syndrome
Oto-palato-digial syndrome
Ruvalcabe syndrome
Conorenal syndrome
Radiation injury

METAPHYSEAL BEAKING

Normal (knees) in bowed legs

Other causes of bowed legs

Epiphyseal metaphyseal fractures in normal bone and battered child syndrome

Blount disease

Epiphyseal metaphyseal fractures in breech delivery

Rickets

Hyperparathyroidism

Neurologic disease

Leukemia, lymphoma

Metastatic disease

Osteomyelitis

Congenital infections

Metabolic bone disease (premature)

Menkes kinky hair syndrome

Scurvy (Pelkan spurs)

Hypophosphatasia

Desbuquis syndrome

ENLARGED VERTEBRAL BODY

1. Paget vertebral body
   * "picture framing"; bone sclerosis
2. Gigantism
   * increase in height of body + disc
3. Myositis ossificans progressiva
   * bodies greater in height than width
   * osteoporosis
   * ossification of ligamentum nuchae

ENLARGED VERTEBRAL FORAMEN

1. Neurofibroma
2. Congenital absence/hypoplasia of pedicle

3. Dural ectasia (Marfan's syndrome, Ehlers-Danlos syndrome)
4. Metastatic destruction of pedicle

STRAIGHTENING OF ANTERIOR BORDER

1. Ankylosing spondylitis
2. Paget's disease
3. Psoriatic arthritis
4. Reiter's disease
5. Rheumatoid arthritis
6. Normal variant

ANTERIOR SCALLOPING OF VERTEBRAE

1. Aortic aneurysm
2. Lymphadenopathy
3. Tuberculosis
4. Multiple myeloma (paravertebral soft tissue mass)

POSTERIOR SCALLOPING OF VERTEBRAE

Mnemonic : "HAMENTS"

Hurler disease, Hydrocephalus

Achondroplasia, Acromegaly

Marfan's syndrome

Ehlers-Danlos syndrome

Tumor (meningioma, ependymoma)

Syringohydromyelia

SPINE OSSIFICATION

A. Syndesmophyte = Ossification of annulus fibrosis associated with : ankylosing spondylitis, ochronosis.

B. Osteophyte

= Ossification of anterior longitudinal ligament, paravertebral soft tissues associated with : diffuse idiopathic skeletal hyperostosis.

C. Flowing anterior ossification

= Ossification of disc, anterior longitudinal ligament, paravertebral soft tissues.

D. Paravertebral ossification

Associated with : psoriatric arthritis, Reiter's disease.

BONE-WITHIN-BONE VERTEBRA

= *"Ghost vertebra"* following stressful event during vertebral growth phase in childhood.

1. Stress line of unknown cause
2. Leukemia
3. Heavy metal poisoning
4. Thorotrast injection
5. Rickets
6. Scurvy
7. Hypothyroidism
8. Hypoparathyroidism

Ivory vertebra

Mnemonic : *"My Only Sister Left Home On Friday Past"*

Myelosclerosis

Osteoblastic metastasis

Sickle-cell disease

Lymphoma

Hemangioma

Osteopetrosis

Fluorosis

Paget's disease

MCQ's ASKED IN VARIOUS ENTRANCE EXAMINATION

MCQ's OF RHEUMATOLOGY

1. **Erb's point is :**
   A. Meeting point of frontal and parietal sutures
   B. Meeting point of anterior division of C5 and C6
   C. At the umbilicus
   D. Meeting point of pleura on left and right side
   E. None of the above
2. **Normal bone remodelling in response to stress was described by :**
   A. Kutschner B. Wolff
   C. Pauwels D. Hugh Owen Thomas
3. **Epiphysis in infant is :**
   A. Cartilage
   B. Calcified
   C. Detected easily by X-ray
   D. Resistant to deformity
4. **Most sensitive structure in a joint is :**
   A. Articular cartilage B. Synovium
   C. Fibrous capsule D. Bone
5. **Bone growth is influenced maximally by :**
   A. Thyroxine B. Growth hormone
   C. Testosterone D. Estrogen
6. **Osteoblasts produce :**
   A. Collagen B. Calcium
   C. Pyrophosphate D. Monosodium urate
7. **The characteristic of collagen is the presence of :**
   A. Glycine B. Methionine
   C. Hydroxyproline D. None of the above

Ans. 1. B 2. B 3. A 4. C 5. B 6. A 7. C

8. **Muscles can withstand arterial occlusion for :**
A. 30 min B. 1 hour
C. 6 hours D. 8 hours

9. **Type of collagen found in cartilage only :**
A. I B. II
C. III D. IV

10. **The tension resistance of normal fascia per square inch, such as the fascia lata, has been determined to be :**
A. 550 pounds B. 1000 pounds
C. 2000 pounds D. 5000 pounds
E. 7000 pounds

11. **A strip of fascia lata 5 mm wide and 0.2 mm thick would have a breaking strength of :**
A. 1/2 pounds B. 5 pounds
C. 10 pounds D. 20 pounds
E. 50 pounds

12. **The safety margin of fascia breaking strength above the physiological stress point is usually :**
A. 20 pounds B. 50 pounds
C. 100 pounds D. 1000 pounds
E. 2000 pounds

13. **Myofibroblast is a cell seen in :**
A. Normal connective tissue
B. Muscle septa
C. Wound margin
D. Lung bronchus

14. **Chondroblast belongs to :**
A. Labile cells B. Stable cells
C. Permanent cells D. All of the above

15. **Longitudial bone growth is dependent on :**
A. Metaphysis B. Diaphysis
C. Epiphysis D. None of the above

16. **The precartilagenous analogue to bone arises from :**
A. Ectoderm B. Entoderm
C. Mesenchyme D. None of the above

Ans. 8. B 9. B 10. E 11. D 12. E 13. C
14. B 15. C 16. C

17. **Cartilage is quite vascular in :**
    A. Embryonic life B. Early childhood
    C. Early adulthood D. Old age

18. **The perichondrial ring is found around :**
    A. Foramen magnum B. Foramina caecum
    C. Epiphyseal plate D. Joint cartilage

19. **The tensile stress resistance of normal tendon per square inch is :**
    A. 550 pounds B. 1000 pounds
    C. 2000 pounds D. 5000 pounds
    E. 7000 pounds

20. **The substance responsible for viscosity of synovial fluid is :**
    A. Chondrotin sulphate B. Heparin sulphate
    C. Hyaluronic acid D. All of the above

21. **Blood supply of bone is :**

	Periosteal	Nutritional
A.	40%	60%
B.	50%	50%
C.	75%	25%
D.	25%	75%

22. **Earliest to ossify in a fetus among the following is :**
    A. Lower end of femur B. Os Calcis
    C. Upper end of tibia D. Mandible

23. **The most radio-sensitive part of the bone is :**
    A. Epiphysis
    B. Osteoblastic layer
    C. Growing cartilage cells
    D. Fibroblasts

24. **True about osteoclast is, except :**
    A. Derived from monocytes
    B. Stimulated by PTH
    C. Phagocytosis of foreign bodies
    D. Resorption of bone

25. **Ossification in foetus starts in :**
    A. 3rd week B. 5th week
    C. 3rd month D. 5th month

Ans. 17. A 18. C 19. D 20. D 21. B 22. D
23. A 24. C 25. B

26. **The true statement regarding bone apposition is :**
    A. Osteoblastic activity in enchondral bone
    B. Chondroblastic activity in enchondral bone
    C. Periosteal cambium layer
    D. Osteoclastic
27. **Decreased activity of osteoblasts is caused by :**
    A. Parathormone B. Vitamin D3
    C. Corticosterone D. T3 and T4
28. **True about synovial fluid are all, except :**
    A. Secreted by Type-A cells
    B. Follows Non-Newtonian fluid kinetics
    C. Contains hyaluronic acid
    D. Viscosity coefficient is variable
29. **Rheumatoid factor is false positive in hepatitis :**
    A. A B. B
    C. C D. D
30. **Increased bone density by X-ray as a result of ischemia may be result of all except :**
    A. Crystalization of fatty acids and the formation of calcium soaps in the infarcted area.
    B. Increased in the thickness of trabeculae.
    C. Fracture and collapse of bone.
    D. Relative disuse atrophy and resorption of the surrounding noninfarcted bone.
    E. Reinforcement of bone in healing or response to stress.
31. **The late radiographic changes seen in active Perthes's disease are all, except :**
    A. Narrow joint space
    B. A widened femoral neck
    C. An irregular density of the epiphysis
    D. An irregular epiphyseal line
    E. A flattened head
32. **Transport media for stones in gout is :**
    A. Distilled water B. Normal saline
    C. Formalin D. Alcohol

Ans. 26. C 27. C 28. A 29. B 30. E 31. A
32. D

33. **Marker for bone formation is :**
A. Osteocalcin
B. Tartarate resistant acid phosphatase
C. 5 nucleotidase
D. Alkaline phosphatase

34. **Bone enzymes found in osteoclasts are :**
A. Acid phosphatases B. Collagenases
C. Glycolytic D. Acid hydrolases
E. All of the above

35. **The radiological features of osteochondritis include :**
A. Mottled density B. Osteoporosis
C. Osteonecrosis D. Attempt at bone repair
E. All of the above

36. **Laboratory findings suggestive of fat embolism in early stages is :**
A. Increase in level of serum fatty acids
B. Lipuria
C. Raised serum alkaline phosphatase
D. Increase in serum lipase

37. **The most confirmatory test for myeloma is :**
A. Aspiration of the lesion and histology
B. Bence-Jones protein in urine
C. Serum electrophoresis
D. Technetium-99 radionuclide bone scan

38. **Epiphyseal enlargement is seen in :**
A. Rheumatoid arthritis B. Still's disease
C. Down's syndrome D. Hypothyroidism

39. **Soft tissue calcification around the knee is seen in :**
A. Scurvy B. Scleroderma
C. Hyperparathyroidism D. Pseudogout

40. **Increased density in metaphysis is seen in :**
A. Hypervitaminosis-D B. Healed rickets
C. Congenital syphilis D. Perthes' disease

41. **Not true about degeneration disease of bone :**
A. Osteophytes B. Decrease in joint space
C. Loose bodies D. Bony ankylosis

Ans. 33. A 34. E 35. E 36. B 37. C 38. B
39. D 40. A 41. D

42. **In osteoporosis, blood picture is :**
    A. ↑ Calcium, ↓ Phosphate, normal alkaline phosphatase
    B. ↓ Calcium, ↑ Phosphate, normal alkaline phosphatase
    C. ↑ Calcium, ↓ Phosphate, ↓ Alkaline phosphatase
    D. Normal
43. **Thurston- Holland sign is present in which type of Salter and Harris type of epiphyseal injury :**
    A. I B. II
    C. III D. IV
    E. V
44. **Diagnostic investigation for bone tumours is :**
    A. FNAC B. Frozen section biopsy
    C. Incisional biopsy D. C.T.
45. **X-ray findings of multiple, spontaneous, idiopathic and symmetrical fractures is characteristic of :**
    A. Stress fracture
    B. Milkman's syndrome
    C. Osteogenesis imperfecta
    D. Osteoporosis
    E. Fluorosis
46. **Which of the following enzymes differentiates osteoclast from osteoblast :**
    A. Alkaline phosphatase B. Acid phosphatase
    C. Deoxyribonuclease D. None of the above
47. **Which of the following is not true regarding synovial fluid :**
    A. Contains HCO_3 and Cl ions more than plasma
    B. Contains mineral ions less than plasma
    C. Contains uric acid more than plasma
    D. Contains fibrinolysin
48. **Which of the following is not found normally in synovial membrane :**
    A. Two layers of lymphatics
    B. Pacinian corpuscles
    C. Basement membrane
    D. A fibrocollagenous layer

Ans. 42. D 43. D 44. C 45. B 46. B 47. C
48. C

49. **False positive rheumatoid factor is present in all, except :**
A. Malaria
B. Leprosy
C. TB
D. Infectious mononucleosis
E. None of the above

50. **C-reactive-protein may be increased in all of the following, except :**
A. Rheumatoid arthritis B. Reactive arthritis
C. SLE related arthritis D. None of the above

51. **The following are radiological features of the haemophilic arthopathy of the knee joint, except :**
A. Widening of the intercondylar notch
B. Epiphyseal overgrowth
C. Increased joint cartilage space
D. Patellar squaring

52. **Mosaic pattern of cement line is characteristically seen in :**
A. Hyperparathyroidism B. Paget's disease of bone
C. Renal osteodystrophy D. Osteomalacia

53. **Synovial fluid has all of the following, except :**
A. Viscid and clear
B. Less than 2,000 cells/cu mm
C. Mucin
D. Fibrinogen

54. **In scaphoid fracture, important views are all, except :**
A. AP B. Lateral
C. Oblique D. Cone

55. **McMurray's sign is positive in injury to :**
A. Medial meniscus
B. Lateral meniscus
C. Anterior cruciate ligament
D. Posterior cruciate ligament

56. **Trendelenburg test +ve in weakness of :**
A. Gluteus maximus B. Gluteus medius
C. Iliopsoas D. Quadratus femoris

Ans. 49. E 50. B 51. C 52. B 53. B 54. D
55. A 56. B

57. **Finckelstein's test is done in :**
A. de Querian's disease
B. Compound palmar ganglia
C. Ulnar nerve palsy
D. Schistosomiasis
E. Fracture scaphoid

58. **X-ray changes in scurvy include :**
A. Pencil line cortex
B. Ringed epiphysis
C. Pathological fractures
D. Widened cupped metaphysis
E. All of the above

59. **Most common joint where arthroscopy is performed is :**
A. Hip
B. Knee
C. Ankle
D. Wrist
E. Elbow

60. **Diagnosis of the osteomyelitis depends on :**
A. X-ray examination
B. Blood culture
C. Clinical examination
D. Urine examination for the presence of albumin

61. **Erosion of bone is seen in all, except :**
A. Osteoarthritis
B. Rheumatoid arthritis
C. Psoriatic arthritis
D. S.L.E

62. **Dead bone is recognised on X-ray because :**
A. It is more radiolucent than normal
B. It is more radiopaque
C. Osteophytes grow out around it
D. It has soap-bubble appearance

63. **Ideal way to do bone biopsy is :**
A. Open biopsy
B. Punch biopsy
C. Needle biopsy
D. None of the above

64. **Physaliphorus cells (large vacuolated cells) on histopathology are characteristic of :**
A. Osteosarcoma
B. Osteoclastoma
C. Liposarcoma
D. Chondrosarcoma
E. Chordoma

Ans. 57. A 58. E 59. B 60. C 61. D 62. B
63. A 64. E

65. **A finding of phosphoethanolamine in the urine is highly suggestive of :**
A. Renal osteodystrophy
B. Hypophosphatasia
C. Hyperparathyroidism
D. Vitamin-D deficiency rickets

66. **Barlow's sign is related to the diagnosis of :**
A. Talipes equinus varus
B. Congenital dislocation of the hip
C. Ulnar nerve palsy
D. Genu venu

67. **Thomas test is done to measure :**
A. Fixed abduction deformity at hip
B. Fixed adduction deformity at hip
C. Fixed flexion deformity at hip
D. Range of rotation at hip

68. **Adson's test involves noticing the :**
A. Pallor in hand
B. Disappearance of radial pulse on the affected side
C. Numbness and tingling on the affected side
D. All of the above

69. **Froment's sign is indicative of :**
A. Lateral popliteal nerve palsy
B. Sciatic nerve palsy
C. Radial nerve palsy
D. Ulnar nerve palsy

70. **Tinel's sign helps in determining regeneration of :**
A. Injured or damaged muscle
B. Injured or sutured nerve
C. Injured or repaired blood vessels
D. None of the above

71. **Phalen's test is positive in :**
A. Tennis elbow
B. de-Quervain's disease
C. Carpal tunnel syndrome
D. Ulnar bursitis

Ans. **65. D** **66. B** **67. C** **68. D** **69. D** **70. B**
71. C

72. **Investigation of choice in traumatic paraplegia is :**
    A. Spine X-ray B. Myelography
    C. CT scan D. MRI
73. **On AP X-ray of hip, abduction of lower limb is denoted by :**
    A. Lesser trochanter obscured by shaft
    B. Greater trochanter is seen fully
    C. Lesser trochanter is seen fully
    D. Lesser sciatic foramen is partly obscured
74. **Antons test is related to :**
    A. Cervical rib
    B. Surgical emphysema
    C. Clavicle fracture
    D. Congenital dislocation of hip
75. **In detecting bone infection, the best ScintiScan agent is :**
    A. 99m TC-MDP B. 67Ga citrate
    C. 111 In-WBC D. All of the above
76. **Capener's sign is positive in :**
    A. Congenital dislocation of hip
    B. Perthes' disease
    C. Adolescent coxa vara
    D. Tuberculous arthritis of hip
77. **'Springing' is a good sign to detect fracture in :**
    A. Humerus B. Femur
    C. Fibula D. Ulna
    E. Tibia
78. **'Ludloff's sign is :**
    A. A prominent lesser trochanter in fracture neck of femur.
    B. When femoral artery is not palpable in posterior dislocation of hip.
    C. Inability to flex the stretched leg in sitting posture in avulsion fracture of lesser trochanter.
    D. Avascular necrosis of the head of femur in fracture neck of femur.
    E. Injury to sciatic nerve in posterior dislocation of hip.

Ans. 72. D 73. C 74. A 75. B 76. C 77. C
78. C

79. **Muscular wasting is a very prominent feature of :**
A. Acute osteomyelitis
B. Chronic osteomyelitis
C. Tuberculous osteomyelitis
D. Syphilitic osteitis
E. Osteomalacia

80. **Presence of Bence Jones protein in the urine though suggestive of multiple myeloma, yet it may also be found in :**
A. Suppurative osteomyelitis
B. Fibrocystic disease
C. Mucopolysaccharide disorders
D. Paget's disease
E. Skeletal carcinomatosis

81. **Cozen's test is :**
A. Inability of the patient to abduct the shoulder.
B. Considerable tenderness at the insertion of supra-spinatus.
C. Patient complains of pain at tip of elbow when he writes.
D. If the patient tries to extend his clenched fist against resistance, pain is experienced at the lateral epicondyle.
E. When the wrist is passively flexed with the forearm pronated pain is complained of at the common extensor origin.

82. **In which condition 'Vascular sign' of Narath will be positive :**
A. Perthes' disease
B. Adolescent coxa vara
C. Congenital dislocation of hip
D. Acute suppurative arthritis
E. Tuberculous arthritis

83. **Kanavel's sign is :**
A. Point of maximum tenderness in case of suppurative tenosynovitis.
B. Maximum tenderness over the medial part of the ulnar bursa between the two transverse palmar creases.
C. Inability to straighten the finger in suppurative tenosynovitis.
D. Maximum tenderness at the proximal end of the bursa round the flexor tendon.
E. Maximum tenderness at the most proximal part of the ulnar bursa.

Ans. 79. C 80. E 81. D 82. C 83. B

84. **Genslen's test is performed to detect the following pathological condition :**
A. Spina bifida
B. Spondylolisthesis
C. Pott's disease
D. Lumbar disc prolapse
E. Sacro-iliac joint pathology

85. **In X-ray the followings from the outline of a 'Scottish Terrier':**
A. The body of the vertebra with pedicles.
B. The body of the vertebral and superior articular facets.
C. The pars interarticularis and the superior articular facets.
D. Pars interarticularis and inferior articular facets.

86. **Cell count greater than 1,00,000/mm^3 in synovial fluid indicates :**
A. Infective arthritis B. Rheumatoid arthritis
C. Gout D. Rheumatoid fever

87. **The 'Card Test' detect the function of :**
A. Median nerve B. Ulnar nerve
C. Axillary nerve D. Radial nerve

88. **An instrument used to measure range of movement around a joint with rheumatoid arthritis is :**
A. Arthrometer B. Goniometer
C. Feleky's instrument D. Hodgen's apparatus

89. **Which is the most sensitive investigation for detecting secondary bony deposits at base of skull :**
A. CT scan B. Radionucleotide scan
C. MRI D. X-ray skull

90. **Raised serum alkaline phosphatase is seen in all except :**
A. Paget's disease B. Multiple myeloma
C. Osteomalacia D. Hyperparathyroidism

91. **Which is the investigation of choice for a sport injury of the knee :**
A. Ultrasonography B. Plain radiography
C. Arthrography D. Arthroscopy

Ans. 84. E 85. C 86. B 87. B 88. B 89. B 90. B 91. D

92. **Bony changes in a case of haematogenous osteomyelitis are earliest seen ——— after the onset.**
A. 10 hours B. 10 days
C. 10 weeks D. 16 weeks

93. **Foot drop is seen in :**
A. Common peroneal nerve injury
B. Tibial nerve injury
C. Achilis tendon injury
D. Popliteal nerve injury

94. **Lachman sign is positive in :**
A. Anterior cruciate ligament injury
B. Posterior cruciate ligament injury
C. Medial meniscus injury
D. Lateral meniscus injury

95. **Following are the causes for nonunion, except :**
A. Systemic illness B. Soft tissue interruption
C. Nerve paralysis D. Haematoma

96. **Mac Nab's sign is most useful in the diagnosis of :**
A. CDH B. Fracture femoral neck
C. Knock knee D. Lumbar spondylosis

97. **In septic arthritis most valuable diagnostic test is :**
A. USS of joint shows bone formation
B. X-ray of the joint
C. Aspiration cytology
D. ESR and blood count study

98. **Earliest detection of Perthes 'disease is by :**
A. Radionuclide scan B. X-ray
C. Clinical examination D. MRI
E. Arthroscopy

99. **Multiple loose bodies are most commonly seen in :**
A. Synovial sarcoma B. Osteoarthritis
C. Perichondritis D. None of the above

100. **In Froment's sign —— muscle is tested.**
A. Adductor pollicis B. Opponens pollicis
C. Flexor pollicis brevis D. Abductor pollicis

Ans. 92. B 93. A 94. A 95. D 96. D 97. C
98. A 99. D 100. A

101. In multiple myeloma, main defect lies in :

A. IgG B. IgM
C. IgA D. IgD

102. In a patient with a tight iliotibial band, the test done is :

A. Charnley's test B. Obson's test
C. Jones' test D. Ober's test

103. Viral osteomyelitis is seen usually to be due vaccination for :

A. Small pox virus infection
B. Influenza virus infection
C. Coxsackie virus infection
D. Dengue fever

104. The definitive treatment for caries spine is :

A. Bed rest
B. Bed rest + antitubercular treatment.
C. Bed rest + antitubercular treatment + drainage of paravertebral abscess.
D. Bed rest + anti-tubercular treatment+drainage of paravertebral abscess and curettage of bony lesion followed by spinal fusion.

105. Caries spine in early stages in a child usually presents as :

A. Pain on sudden motion B. Lumbar lordosis
C. Night cries D. Gibbus formation

106. Chances of paraplegia are maximum in caries of :

A. Cervical spine B. Upper thoracic spine
C. Dorso-lumbar spine D. Lumbar spine

107. Complications of osteomyelitis include all, except :

A. Pathological fracture B. Amyloidosis
C. Septicemia D. Malignancy

108. Which of the following is not true regarding Brodie's abscess :

A. It is a type of chronic osteomyelitis.
B. Small sequestra are usually present in the cavity.
C. It is present in epiphyseal part of bone.
D. It is cavity surrounded by densely sclerosed bone.

Ans. 101. A 102. D 103. A 104. D 105. A 106. C
107. D 108. C

109. **HIV osteomylitis, true is :**
A. B/L lesions
B. Caused by Staph aureus
C. New bone formation not seen
D. Necrosis not seen

110. **Earliest radiological finding of TB spine is :**
A. Collapse of vertebra
B. Narrowing of disc space
C. Cold abscess formation
D. Pedicle shadow erosion

111. **T.B. hip commonly starts in :**
A. Babcock's triangle B. Scarpa's triangle
C. Petit's triangle D. None of the above

112. **Osteomyelitis of one week duration is treated by :**
A. Drainage & appropriate antibiotic
B. Antibiotic and plaster immobilisation
C. Antibiotic and traction
D. Antibiotic and blood transfusion

113. **Tuberculous arthritis in advanced cases lead to :**
A. Bony ankylosis B. Fibrous ankylosis
C. Loose joints D. Charcot's joints

114. **Acute hematogenous osteomyelitis is treated with all, except :**
A. Antibiotics B. Splinting
C. Analgesics D. Surgery

115. **Earliest manifestation of spinal TB is :**
A. Cold abscess formation B. Paraplegia
C. Gibbus D. Muscle spasm

116. **Commonest organism causing osteomyelitis in children under 3 years is :**
A. Hemophilus B. Staphylococcal
C. Streptococcal D. Salmonella

117. **Commonest site for acute osteomyelitis in infant is :**
A. Hip joint B. Tibia
C. Femur D. Radial

Ans. 109. B 110. B 111. A 112. A 113. B 114. D
115. D 116. A 117. A

118. False about capsulitis in shoulder is :
A. Prolonged immobility lead to it
B. Tenderness at shoulder
C. Tenderness on abduction
D. Tenderness on passive movements

119. Extensive curettage is contraindicated if osteomyelitis is located in :
A. Calcaneus
B. Tibia
C. Fibula
D. Ribs

120. Organism found in chronic osteomyelitis is :
A. Staph. aureus
B. Staph. pyogenus
C. E. coli
D. Staph. epidermitis

121. Hematogenous osteomyelitis is seen in which part of the bone:
A. Epiphysis
B. Metaphysis
C. Diaphysis
D. Area of nutrient artery distribution

122. True about acute suppurative arthritis is all, except :
A. May be caused by a penetrating wound.
B. May be caused by a compound fracture involving a joint.
C. May be due to blood-borne infection with the gonococcus.
D. Causes the joint to be held in the position of ease.
E. Tends to end with the formation of a fibrous ankylosis.

123. Bone lesions in syphilis are following except :
A. Periarthritis
B. Periosteitis
C. Osteomyelitis
D. Charcot's joint

124. Tertiary syphilitic arthritis most frequently involves :
A. Spine
B. Hip
C. Ankle
D. Knee
E. Shoulder

125. The most frequent offending agent in osteomyelitis of the spine is :
A. Streptococcus
B. Salmonella
C. Pneumococcus
D. E. coli
E. Tubercle bacillus

Ans. 118. D 119. A 120. A 121. D 122. A 123. D
124. E 125. D

126. **Which of the following terms is inappropriate to the condition osteomyelitis :**
A. Cloaca B. Involucrum
C. Sequestrum D. Myelocele

127. **Psoas spasm is seen in the following :**
A. TB hip
B. TB spine
C. Ac. appendicitis
D. Mesenteric iliac lymphadenitis

128. **Pott's disease is :**
A. A fracture dislocation about the ankle
B. A neuropathic joint
C. Traumatic osteochondritis of the spine
D. Tuberculous of the spine

129. **Swollen appearance in a case of tuberculosis knee is due to :**
A. Synovial thickening B. Local oedema
C. Muscle wasting D. Abscess formation
E. Dislocation of joint

130. **Tuberculous infection in spine settles down in :**
A. Nucleus pulposus
B. Intervertebral ligaments
C. Cancellous vertebral body
D. Paravertebral muscles

131. **Diffuse systemic osteoarthritis is seen in the following, except :**
A. Ankle joint B. CMP
C. Elbow D. DIP

132. **Erosive arthritis is seen in all, except :**
A. Gout B. Osteoarthritis
C. SLE D. Hyperparathyroidism

133. **Acute infection in tendon sheath of ring finger can spread to:**
A. Mid palmar crease B. Space of Perona
C. Elbow D. Thumb

134. **Acute osteomyelitis of the following site is likely to spread to the adjacent joint :**
A. Upper end of humerus B. Upper end of tibia
C. Upper end of femur D. Lower end of femur

Ans. 126. A 127. D 128. A 129. C 130. C 131. C
132. A 133. C 134. A

135. **The most commonly affected lower limb muscle in poliomyelitis is :**
A. Quadriceps femoris B. Tibialis anterior
C. Tibialis posterior D. Peroneus longus

136. **Spinal tuberculosis is most common in :**
A. The cervical region B. Upper dorsal region
C. Lower dorsal region D. Lumborsacral region

137. **When does the lesion of osteomyelitis appear in X-rays :**
A. 2 hours B. 24 hours
C. 1 week D. 2 weeks

138. **TB of joint, features are all, except :**
A. Synovium is involved
B. Synovium fluid has < 20% blood sugar
C. Kissing arthritis-subchondral involved
D. Pain is common feature
E. None of the above

139. **The treatment of osteomyelitis is :**
A. Antibiotics B. Saucerization
C. A + B of the above D. Amputation

140. **In septic arthritis, most diagnostic is :**
A. Arthrocentesis B. Peripheral smear
C. ESR D. None of the above

141. **In hand infection, true is following, except :**
A. Elevation and rest B. Incision and drainage
C. X-ray to locate incision D. Antibiotics
E. Trauma usual cause

142. **Osteomyelitis of jaw is seen in :**
A. Caffey's disease B. Osteomalacia
C. Osteoporosis D. Osteopoikilosis

143. **Osteomyelitis of skull commonly follows :**
A. Fracture base of skull B. Paranasal sinus infection
C. Dental sepsis D. Ear injection

144. **Syphilitic osteoperiostitis is most common in :**
A. Femur B. Tibia
C. Humerus D. Spine

Ans. 135. C 136. D 137. D 138. C 139. A 140. C
141. A 142. B 143. B 144. C

145. The ideal treatment for osteomyelitis is :
A. Prolonged antibiotic therapy
B. Curettage
C. Saucerization and antibiotics
D. Bed rest

146. All of the following are seen in inflammatory polyarthritis, except :
A. Spontaneous flares
B. ↑ ESR
C. New bone formation
D. Morning stiffness more than 30 minutes

147. Tom Smith arthritis involves :
A. Head of femur
B. Knee joint
C. Head of humerus
D. Elbow

148. Polio paralysis differs from paralysis due to other causes by :
A. Weakness of muscles
B. Deformity of limbs
C. No sensory loss
D. Full recovery is possible

149. Commonest cause of osteomyelitis in HbS disease is :
A. Staph. aureus
B. Streptococcus
C. Pneumococcus
D. Salmonella

150. The dead bone seen in chronic osteomyelitis is called :
A. Sequestrum
B. Involucrum
C. Sinus debris
D. Cloaca

151. Commonest type of spinal tuberculosis is :
A. Anterior
B. Paradiscal
C. Pedicle
D. Posterior

152. First symptom of TB spine is :
A. Decreased motor power
B. Decreased sensations
C. ↓ deep tendon reflexes
D. Pain

153. Commonest site for TB bone after spine is :
A. Hip
B. Knee
C. Shoulder
D. Ankle

154. Regarding Tom Smith Arthritis, not true is :
A. May lead to bony ankylosis
B. Affected limb is usually shorter in length
C. Seen mainly in infants
D. Associated with epigastric septic adenoma

Ans. 145. C 146. A 147. D 148. D 149. A 150. B
151. D 152. A 153. D 154. A

155. **Painless effusion in joints in congenital syphilis is called :**
A. Clutton's joints
B. Barton's patients
C. Charcot's joints
D. Synovitis

156. **Sequestrum is a :**
A. Infected bone
B. New bone
C. Dead bone
D. Woven bone

157. **Ring sequestrum is seen in :**
A. Infected amputated stump
B. Chr. osteomyelitis
C. Osteosarcoma
D. TB spine

158. **Tom-Smith arthritis spreads to the hip joint because :**
A. Metaphysis is inside the joint
B. Epiphysis is absent
C. Periosteum lacks a cambium layer
D. All of the above

159. **The etiology of Tom-Smith arthritis is :**
A. Pyogenic
B. Rheumatoid
C. Fungal
D. Syphilis

160. **Equinus deformity in polio is due to weakness of :**
A. Invertors
B. Dorsi flexors
C. Plantar flexors
D. Evertors

161. **A case of poliomyelitis has the following power- grades in his lower limb gastrosoleus grade-I, tibialis anterior grade-IV, peroneus-III and power around the knee and hip are normal. The most likely deformity he will develop is :**
A. Talipes
B. Calcaneus
C. Calcaneovalgus
D. Equinovalgus

162. **Tuberculosis of hip presents with very characteristic deformities in various stages of the disease. The deformities in the 3rd stage of tuberculosis of hip include flexion :**
A. Adduction and internal rotation
B. Adduction and external rotation
C. Abduction and external rotation
D. Abduction and internal rotation

Ans. 155. C 156. B 157. A 158. A 159. D
160. B 161. D 162. A

163. **Bone marrow tuberculosis shows :**
A. Leucoerythroblastic change
B. AFB +ve
C. Thrombocytosis
D. Eosinophilia

164. **Early features of spinal tuberculosis in a child is :**
A. Night cries
B. Sudden deformity
C. Gradual deformity
D. Pain on sudden movement

165. **A leprosy patient experiences clumsiness of hand, the lesion lies in ulnar nerve and it is due to palsy of :**
A. Interosseous muscle
B. Extensor carpi ulnaris
C. Abductor pollicis
D. Opponens pollicis

166. **In a post-polio case, ilio-tibial tract contracture is likely to result in :**
A. Extension at the hip and knee
B. Extension at the hip
C. Flexion at the hip and the knee
D. Extension at the knee

167. **In a 15-years old boy with an expansile lytic lesion in the upper part of humerus with one side of cortex broken. The most likely diagnosis is :**
A. Unicameral bone cyst
B. Aneurysmal bone cyst
C. Chondroblastoma
D. Osteoclastoma

168. **Treatment of choice for cystic tuberculosis of bone is :**
A. Chemotherapy only
B. Curettage & chemotherapy
C. Radiotherapy
D. Amputation

169. **In actinomycosis of the spine, the abscess usually erodes :**
A. Intervertebral disc
B. Into the pleural cavity
C. Into the retroperitoneal space
D. Towards the skin

170. **Which group of muscles is most commonly affected in poliomyelitis :**
A. Dorsiflexors of the ankle
B. Flexors of the knee
C. Flexors of the hip
D. Extensors of the hip

Ans. 163. A 164. A 165. A 166. C 167. A 168. B
169. D 170. A

171. The joint most often affected by osteoarthritis is :
A. Spine B. Hip
C. Knee D. Ankle

172. Long-term follow-up studies show the incidence of osteoarthritis in the closed treatment of simple posterior dislocation (Epstein grade-1) to be :
A. Less than 5% B. Less than 10%
C. Less than 20% D. Less than 40%

173. Osteoarthrosis in triple fusion is commonest at joint of :
A. Talonavicular B. Calcaneocuboid
C. Talocalcaneal D. Naviculocuboid

174. Primary osteoarthritis is not found in :
A. Hip
B. Shoulder
C. Spine
D. 1st metatarsophalangeal joint

175. Treatment of osteoarthritis include all, except :
A. Graded muscle exercises
B. Replacement of articular surfaces
C. Correction of deformities
D. Increase the weight bearing by the affected joint
E. Rest to the joint in acute phase

176. Drug of choice in juvenile chronic arthritis in children is :
A. Aspirin B. Indomethacin
C. Prednisolone D. Phenylbutazone

177. Osteoarthritis following is not a predisposing factor :
A. Diabetes mellitus B. Defective joint position
C. Weight bearing joints D. Incongruity of articular surfaces
E. Old age

178. Treatment of osteoarthritis include following, except :
A. Graded muscle exercises
B. Replacement of articular surfaces
C. Correction of deformities
D. Increase the weight bearing by the affected joint
E. Rest to the joint in acute phase

Ans. 171. B 172. C 173. C 174. B 175. D 176. A
177. A 178. D

179. Osteoarthritis of knee causes :
A. ↑ Flexion
B. - Extension
C. Varus deformity
D. Valgus deformity

180. All of the following are found in shoulder joint osteoarthritis, except :
A. Subchondral sclerosis
B. Osteophytes in humeral head
C. Osteochondral fragmentation
D. Joint space narrowed

181. Osteoarthritis occurs at an early age in :
A. Ehler Danlos syndrome
B. Marfan's syndrome
C. Hurler syndrome
D. Fabry's disease

182. The common sites in the hip region that are affected by tuberculosis are the following, except :
A. Acetabular roof
B. Lesser trochanter
C. Head of femur
D. Neck of femur
E. Greater trochanter

183. The earliest change in osteoarthritis is :
A. Eburnation
B. Fibrillation of cartilage
C. Loose bodies
D. Subchondral microcysts

184. The rheumatoid nodule is found in the following except :
A. Kidney
B. Lungs
C. Pleura
D. Dura mater

185. The cause of rheumatoid arthritis is :
A. Heredity
B. Immunological
C. Infective
D. Traumatic

186. Rheumatoid Arthritis - anaemia, true is :
A. Normocytic normochromic
B. Macrocytic
C. Microcytic
D. Associated with thrombocytosis

187. Remission inducing drugs or disease modifying drugs for Rheumatoid arthritis include :
A. Aspirin
B. Iburpofen
C. Gold Thiol
D. Neproxan

Ans. 179. A 180. C 181. A 182. B 183. B 184. A
185. B 186. A 187. C

188. Treatment of rheumatoid arthritis include all, except :
A. Give rest to the joint B. Correction of deformities
C. Synovectomy D. Exercises
E. Drugs immuno-suprasive

189. The type of pericarditis seen in rheumatoid arthritis is :
A. Fibrinous B. Serofibrinous
C. Purulent D. Serous

190. Rheumatoid factor is most commonly positive in :
A. SLE
B. Sjogren's syndrome
C. Adult Rheumatoid arthritis
D. Sarcoidosis

191. In rheumatoid arthritis, pathology starts in :
A. Articular cartilage B. Synovia
C. Capsule D. Muscles

192. Consider the following manifestations :
1. Keratoconjunctivitis sicca
2. Hearing impairment
3. Hoarseness of voice
4. Pericarditis

Extra-articular manifestations of rheumatoid arthritis would include :
A. 1, 2, 3 and 4 B. 1, 3 and 4
C. 2, 3 and 4 D. 1 and 2

193. Which of the following may lead to Charcot's joint :
A. Tabes dorsalis B. Peripheral neuritis
C. Syringomyelia D. Any of the above

194. Melon seed bodies are characteristic of :
A. Tubercular arthritis B. Rheumatoid arthritis
C. Syphilitic arthritis D. Charcot's joint
E. Osteoarthritis

195. Bony ankylosis is noticed in cases of :
A. Tubercular arthritis B. Pyogenic arthritis
C. Rheumatoid arthritis D. None of the above

Ans. 188. A 189. A 190. B 191. B 192. B 193. D
194. A 195. B

196. Ankylosing spondylitis involve the following, except :
A. Spine and Hip B. Sacroiliac joint
C. Elderly D. Hypermobility

197. Carpal tunnel syndrome is seen in all, except :
A. Pregnancy B. Hypothyroidism
C. Knee D. Wrist and Elbow

198. Bamboo spine is seen in :
A. Ankylosing spondylosis
B. Rheumatoid arthritis
C. Scheurmann's disease
D. Pott's spine

199. Pain in Paget's disease is best relieved by :
A. Simple analgesics B. Narcotic analgesics
C. Radiation D. Calcitonin

200. Senile osteoporosis radiologically manifest only when ——— of skeleton has been lost.
A. 20% B. 30%
C. 40% D. 80%

201. The complication of Paget's disease is :
A. Osteogenic sarcoma B. Deafness
C. Heart failure D. All of the above

202. In gout arthritis, following are true, except :
A. Urate crystals
B. Joint space reduced
C. Great toe commonly affected
D. Serum uric acid useful test

203. All are characteristics of osteoarthritis, except :
A. Early morning stiffness lasting for about 30 minutes
B. E.S.R > 30 mm at the end of 1st hour
C. Widening of the joint space
D. Focal degeneration of articular cartilage is seen

204. Osteochondromatosis most often involves :
A. Hip B. Shoulder
C. Ankle D. Elbow

Ans. 196. D 197. C 198. A 199. D 200. C 201. D
202. B 203. B 204. A

205. Osteochondritis dissecans is characterized by all except :
A. Common in sportsman
B. Bilateral in 75%
C. Knee commonest involved
D. 'Locking or sensation, of giving away common

206. In which of the following manifestations of osteomyelitis, the pathological fracture is more common :
A. Brodies abscess
B. Sclerosing osteomyelitis
C. Subacute stage of osteomyelitis
D. Chronic osteomyelitis

207. Winging of scapula is caused by :
A. Serratus anterior palsy
B. Lattismus dorsi involvement
C. Deltoid muscle palsy
D. Brachioradialis

208. Frost-bite arthritis is similar to :
A. Osteoarthritis
B. Rheumatoid arthritis
C. Psoriatic arthritis
D. Ankylosing spondylitis

209. Ankylosing spondylitis involves first of all :
A. Hip joint
B. Sacroiliac joint
C. Spine
D. Shoulder joint

210. What do you understand by the term'Meralgia paresthetica' :
A. Complete anaesthesia along the distribution of median nerve.
B. Complete anaesthesia along the paravertebral muscles.
C. Hypesthesias and Dysesthesia in the cutaneous distribution of lateral femoral cutaneous nerve.
D. None of the above.

211. Neuropathic joint may arise in :
A. Syringomyelia
B. Tabes dorsalis
C. Leprosy
D. All of the above

212. The early X-ray changes of ankylosing spondylitis would be:
A. Disc space narrowing
B. Anterior osteophyte formation
C. Sacroiliac joint erosion
D. Facetal joint ankylosis

Ans. 205. B 206. D 207. A 208. B 209. B 210. C
211. D 212. C

213. **Dupuytren's contracture most commonly involves :**
A. Fourth finger B. Fifth finger
C. Fourth and fifth fingers D. Thumb and forefinger

214. **Match List—I (type of diseases commonly seen in orthopaedic O.P.D) with List-II (choice of treatment for the concerned disease) and select the correct answer using the codes given below the lists :**

List -I	List -II
A. Osteoarthritis of the knee	1. Long leg pop cast
B. Friction type bursa on anterior aspect of knee	2. Local hydrocortisone
C. Haemophilia with involvement of knee	3. Pressure bandage
D. Tuberculous synovitis of knee	4. Quadriceps exercises
	5. Aspiration + pressure bandage

Codes :

	A	B	C	D
A.	2	3	5	4
B.	4	2	5	1
C.	3	4	5	1
D.	4	2	3	1

215. **The intervertebral distance is reduced in the following :**
A. Compression of the vertebra
B. Multiple myeloma
C. Caries spine
D. All of the above

216. **True about Perthes's disease is :**
A. Common in boys B. Common in girls
C. Common in elderly D. Common in all age groups

Ans. 213. C 214. C 215. C 216. A

217. A paralysed bladder following spinal injury is best managed by :
A. Foley's catheter B. Gibbson's catheter
C. Metallic catheter D. Malicot catheter

218. Gradually increasing stiffness of shoulder is seen in :
A. Rheumatoid arthritis B. Periarthrosis
C. Osteoarthritis D. Reiter's disease

219. The following are radiological signs of Paget's disease of bone except :
A. "Cotton Wool" appearance
B. "Picture Window Frame" appearance
C. "Hair-on-end" appearance
D. "Blade of grass" appearance

220. Positivity of HLA B 27 in ankylosing spondylosis :
A. 10% B. 96%
C. 78% D. 100%
E. Ankle - at a right angle

221. Triple deformity of knee is seen in :
A. Tuberculosis B. Patella
C. Rheumatoid arthritis D. Rheumatic arthritis

222. Anserine bursitis is seen in :
A. OA B. RA
C. SLE D. Psoriatic

223. Bursitis in origin may be :
A. Traumatic B. Pyogenic
C. Gonococcal D. Syphilitic
E. Any of the above

224. Rugzer Jersy sign is present in :
A. Ankylosing spondylitis B. TB spine
C. Osteoarthritis D. Myeloma
E. C/C renal failure

225. 'Paget's disease' is also known by the name of :
A. Osteitis fibrosa cystica B. Osteitis proliferans
C. Osteitis deformans D. Osteitis pubis

Ans. 217. A 218. B 219. C 220. B 221. A 222. B
223. E 224. A 225. C

226. **The level of serum calcium in cases of Paget's disease is :**
    A. Normal (Unchanged)
    B. Decreased
    C. Increased
    D. Changed according to serum alkaline phosphatase level
227. **Osteoporosis in India is noticed commonly due to :**
    A. Gonadal deficiency
    B. Pituitary hormone deficiency
    C. Trauma
    D. Senility
228. **Regarding Paget's disease of bone, which of the following is not true :**
    A. Males are affected more than females.
    B. Serum alkaline phosphatase is low.
    C. Involved area shows rapid formation and resorption of bone.
    D. It frequently leads to osteogenic sarcoma.
229. **The histopathologic feature of Paget's disease include :**
    A. Osteoclastic resorption.
    B. Replacement of bone marrow by fibrovascular tissue.
    C. Simultaneous osteoclastic and osteoblastic activity at place.
    D. All of the above.
    E. None of the above.
230. **Regarding Paget's disease :**
    A. Commonly occurs in middle age
    B. May be monostotic or polyostotic
    C. May produce some neurological symptoms
    D. Affected bones may be develop osteogenic sarcoma secondarily
    E. All of the above are true
231. **Median nerve supplies all the following, except :**
    A. Pronator teres
    B. Flexor carpi radialis
    C. Pronator quadratus
    D. 1st and 2nd lumbricals
    E. 3rd and 4th lumbricals
232. **Causalgia usually affects :**
    A. Radial nerve
    B. Median nerve
    C. Ulnar nerve
    D. Circumflex humeral nerve

Ans. 226. A 227. D 228. B 229. D 230. E 231. E
232. B

233. **Acute osteomyelitis is most common in :**
A. Upper end of tibia
B. Upper end of femur
C. Lower end of femur
D. Upper end of humerus

234. **In Gout, the crystals are :**
A. Calcium pyrophosphate
B. Monosodium urate
C. Monopotassium urate
D. Double phosphate

235. **Which of the following is not a cause of osteoporosis :**
A. Calcium deficiency
B. Phosphate deficiency
C. Prolonged immobilization
D. Steroid intake

236. **The most effective drug for seronegative ankylosing spondylitis is :**
A. Aspirin B. Corticosteroids
C. Indomethacin D. Pencillamine

237. **FISH-vertebra is a feature of :**
A. Paget's disease B. Fragilates ossium
C. Osteomalacia D. All of the above

238. **Severance of the ulnar nerve at the wrist causes :**
A. Loss of sensation on the anterior and posterior aspects of the inner one and a half fingers.
B. Inability to flex the terminal phalanx of the little finger.
C. Flexion of the little finger at the metacarpophalangeal joint.
D. Inability to abduct or adduct the fingers.
E. A positive Froment's sign.

239. **Volkman's ischemia most commonly involves :**
A. Pronator teres
B. Flexor carpii radialis longus
C. Flexor digitorum profundus
D. Flexor digitorum superficials

Ans. 233. C 234. B 235. B 236. C 237. D 238. A
239. C

240. **Most common cause of Tardy ulnar nerve palsy is :**
    A. Supracondylar fracture
    B. Fracture of lateral condyle
    C. Posterior elbow dislocation
    D. Fracture of olecranon
241. **Axillary nerve injury at its origin leads to paralysis of :**
    A. Deltoid & teres minor   B. Deltoid
    C. Deltoid & teres major   D. Lattismus dorsi and deltoid
242. **In Sedden's classification, complete division of nerve is :**
    A. Neuropraxia   B. Axonotemesis
    C. Neurotemesis   D. None of the above
243. **Peripheral nerves can resist ischemia upto :**
    A. 30 minutes   B. 1 hour
    C. 6 hours   D. 12 hours
244. **Earliest symptom of Volkman's ischemia is :**
    A. Pain in flexor muscles
    B. Absence of pulse
    C. Pain on passive extension
    D. Cyanosis of limb
245. **Most common cause of Neuropathic joints is :**
    A. Leprosy   B. Diabetes
    C. Rheumatoid arthritis   D. Syphilis
246. **Avascular necrosis of bone is most commcnly seen in :**
    A. Calcaneus   B. Cervical spine
    C. Scaphoid   D. Scapula
247. **Congenital pseudoarthrosis is seen in :**
    A. Tibia-Fibula   B. Femur
    C. Femur-Tibia   D. Hip joint
248. **Dissociative sensory loss is seen in :**
    A. Tabes dorsalis   B. Syringomyelia
    C. Disc prolapse   D. T.B. spine
249. **Phantom limb is an example of :**
    A. Topographic dislocation
    B. Weber's law
    C. Wrong projection due to incorrect localization nerve
    D. Law of specific nerve energies

Ans. 240. B 241. A 242. C 243. B 244. A 245. B
246. C 247. A 248. B 249. C

250. **Johnson-Larsen's disease is osteochondritis of :**
   A. Capital femoral epiphysis
   B. Lunate bone
   C. Navicular bone
   D. Tibial tubercle
   E. Lower pole of the patella
251. **A young man with backache and asymmetric lower limb weakness has :**
   A. Seronegative spondylosis
   B. Rheumatoid arthritis
   C. OA
   D. Gout
252. **In case of paralysis of the intrinsic muscles of the hand with 'main-en-griffe', the lesion is at :**
   A. C4 B. C6
   C. C7 D. T1
   E. T2
253. **Radial nerve injury of which type recovers with conservative management :**
   A. Neurotemesis B. Crush injury
   C. Neuropraxia D. Chemical injury
254. **Injury to ulnar nerve at wrist causes paralysis of :**
   A. Opposition of thumb
   B. Abduction at CMC joint or thumb
   C. Adduction of thumb
   D. Flexion of MCP joint of thumb
255. **Which one of the following does not involve nerve damage :**
   A. Erb's paralysis B. Gullain-Barre syndrome
   C. Volkman's paralysis D. Neurotemesis
256. **Injury to ulnar nerve at wrist causes paralysis of :**
   A. Opposition of thumb
   B. Abduction at CMC joint of thumb
   C. Adduction of thumb
   D. Flexion of MCP joint of middle finger

Ans. **250. E 251. A 252. D 253. C 254. C 255. C 256. C**

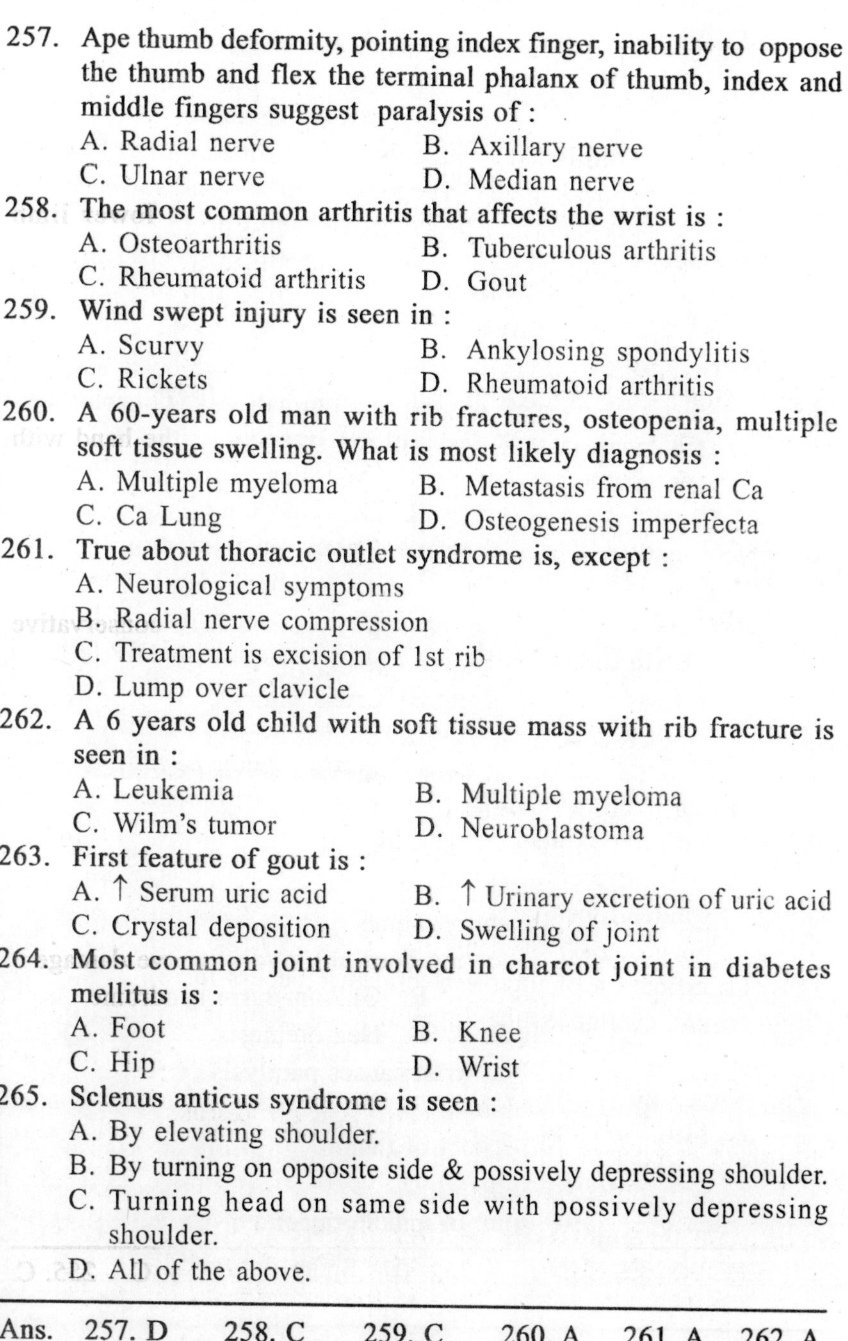

257. Ape thumb deformity, pointing index finger, inability to oppose the thumb and flex the terminal phalanx of thumb, index and middle fingers suggest paralysis of :
   A. Radial nerve B. Axillary nerve
   C. Ulnar nerve D. Median nerve

258. The most common arthritis that affects the wrist is :
   A. Osteoarthritis B. Tuberculous arthritis
   C. Rheumatoid arthritis D. Gout

259. Wind swept injury is seen in :
   A. Scurvy B. Ankylosing spondylitis
   C. Rickets D. Rheumatoid arthritis

260. A 60-years old man with rib fractures, osteopenia, multiple soft tissue swelling. What is most likely diagnosis :
   A. Multiple myeloma B. Metastasis from renal Ca
   C. Ca Lung D. Osteogenesis imperfecta

261. True about thoracic outlet syndrome is, except :
   A. Neurological symptoms
   B. Radial nerve compression
   C. Treatment is excision of 1st rib
   D. Lump over clavicle

262. A 6 years old child with soft tissue mass with rib fracture is seen in :
   A. Leukemia B. Multiple myeloma
   C. Wilm's tumor D. Neuroblastoma

263. First feature of gout is :
   A. ↑ Serum uric acid B. ↑ Urinary excretion of uric acid
   C. Crystal deposition D. Swelling of joint

264. Most common joint involved in charcot joint in diabetes mellitus is :
   A. Foot B. Knee
   C. Hip D. Wrist

265. Sclenus anticus syndrome is seen :
   A. By elevating shoulder.
   B. By turning on opposite side & possively depressing shoulder.
   C. Turning head on same side with possively depressing shoulder.
   D. All of the above.

Ans. 257. D 258. C 259. C 260. A 261. A 262. A
263. A 264. A 265. B

266. Ossification of interossous membrane is seen in :
A. Osteopetrosis
B. Vit. A intoxication
C. Fluorosis
D. All of the above

267. A 66 years old female with compressed fracture of T11 vertebra had hypocalcemia, hypophosphatemia and raised serum alkaline phosphatase. The diagnosis could be :
A. Osteoporosis
B. Paget's disease of bone
C. Primary hyperparathyroidism
D. Rickets

268. Serum Ca++ normal, phosphorus normal, Alk. phosphatase 3 times normal, in a 67 years old, disease is :
A. Osteomalacia
B. Metastatic bone lesion
C. Paget's disease
D. Lead poisoning

269. Neuropathic joint of foot and ankle - most common :
A. Hansen
B. Mycetoma
C. CTEV
D. Polio

270. Hyperextension of PIP joint and hyperflexion of DIP joints, is known as :
A. Swan neck deformity
B. Boutonnieri deformity
C. Mallet finger
D. Carpal Tunnel syndrome

271. Which is not a feature of Dupuytren's contracture :
A. Recurrent trauma
B. Genetic predilection
C. Bilateral lesions rare
D. Seen equally in males and females

272. Calcification of inter-vertebral disc occurs in :
A. Ankylosing spondylitis
B. Alkaptonuria
C. Osteomalacia
D. Neurofibroma

273. Ring sign is seen in :
A. Osteosarcoma
B. Osteoclastoma
C. Rickets
D. Barlow's disease

274. Spina ventosa is caused by :
A. Tuberculosis
B. Leprosy
C. Metastasis
D. Spine deformity

Ans. 266. C 267. A 268. C 269. A 270. A 271. D
272. B 273. C, D 274. A

275. **Which among the following should not be given in acute gout :**
A. Acetyl salicylic acid B. Indomethacin
C. Piroxicam D. Allopurinol

276. **Dupuytren's contracture, true is :**
A. Dermal contracture
B. Common in males
C. Early sign is palmar nodule
D. Common in orientals

277. **Calcification around joint is seen in :**
A. Alkaptonuria B. Hyperparathyroidism
C. Pseudohypothyroidism D. Pseudogout

278. **Erosion of hyaline cartilage is seen in all except :**
A. RA B. Gout
C. SLE D. Psoriasis

279. **'Painfull arc syndrome' is a clinical condition of the shoulder in which the middle range of the arc of abduction is painful. Which one of the following is not a cause of this condition :**
A. Rupture of the supraspinatus tendon
B. Supraspinatus tendinitis
C. Acromioclavicular arthritis
D. Subacromial bursitis

280. **Osteosclerotic bone lesions are seen in all, except :**
A. Multiple myeloma B. Metastasis
C. Spina ventasa D. Fluorosis

281. **Bibrachial palsy leads to :**
A. Wrist drop B. Dangling arm
C. Extension of arm D. Hyperkinetic movements

282. **In a patient with 4 days old acute compartment syndrome, treatment of choice is :**
A. Debridement B. Amputation
C. Foot drop splint D. Fasciotomy

283. **Collapse and fragmentation of lunate bone is which stage of Kienbock's disease :**
A. I B. II
C. III D. IV

Ans. 275. D 276. C 277. D 278. C 279. C 280. A
281. B 282. B 283. C

284. Following are causes of rigid flat foot, except :
A. Osteoarthritis
B. Rheumatoid arthritis
C. Spastic peroneal foot
D. Tarsal coalition

285. In painful syndrome, all of the following lesions can be found, except :
A. Subacromial bursitis
B. Complete tear of supraspinatus
C. Fracture of the greater tubercle
D. Rotator cuff injury

286. Sclerotic bones are found in all the following, except :
A. Pagets' disease
B. Osteopetrosis
C. Osteoporosis
D. Metastasis

287. A 4½-years old girl always had to warm socks even in summer season. On physical examination, it was noticed that she had high blood pressure and her femoral pulse was weak as compared to radial and carotid pulse. A chest radiograph showed remarkable notching of ribs along with their lower borders. This was due to :
A. Femoral artery thrombosis
B. Coarctation of aorta
C. Raynaud's disease
D. Takayasu's arthritis

288. Kienbock's disease is due to avascular necrosis of :
A. Femoral neck
B. Medial cuneiform
C. Lunate bone
D. Scaphoid bone

289. Avascular necrosis can be a possible sequela of fracture of all the following bones, except :
A. Femur neck
B. Scaphoid
C. Talus
D. Calcaneum

290. A 10 years old girl presents with swelling of one knee joint. All of the following conditions can be considered in the differential diagnosis, except :
A. Tuberculosis
B. Juvenile rheumatoid arthritis
C. Haemophilia
D. Vilonodular synovitis

Ans. 284. A 285. B 286. C 287. B 288. C 289. D 290. C

291. In osteomalacia the cause of softing of the bones is which of the following :
    A. Decreasing in osteoid volume
    B. Decrease in osteoid surface
    C. Increase in osteoid maturation time
    D. Increase in mineral aposition rate

292. The classical flexion and rotation deformities at hip and knee joints, as a sequela of poliomyelitis, are due to the contracture of :
    A. Tensor facia lata B. Gastrocnemius
    C. Tendon achilles D. Hamstrings

293. Avascular necrosis is seen in all of the following, except :
    A. Upper end of humerus B. Body of talus
    C. Head of femur D. Scapula

294. Tuberculosis of the spine commonly affects all of the following parts of the vertebra, except:
    A. Body B. Lamina
    C. Spinous process D. Pedicle

295. An army recruit, smoker and 6 months into training started complaining of pain at posterior medial aspect of both legs. There was acute point tenderness and the pain was aggravated on physical activity. The most likely diagnosis is:
    A. Buerger's disease B. Gout
    C. Lumbar canal stenosis D. Stress fracture

296. All the following are true of primary sub acute osteomyelitis except :
    A. Brodie's abscess
    B. Garre's osteomyelitis
    C. Salmonella osteomyelitis
    D. Brucellar osteomyelitis

297. The most common cause for anterior knee pain is :
    A. Prepatellar bursitis
    B. Congenital discoid meniscus
    C. Plica syndrome
    D. Chondromalaria patellae

Ans. 291. C 292. A 293. D 294. C 295. D 296. D 297. D

298. **Angular kyphosis is most commonly produced by :**
A. Rickets
B. Senile osteoporosis
C. Tuberculosis of spine
D. Hyperparathyroidism

299. **Congenital constriction ring of the leg is treated by :**
A. Excision and resuture
B. Excision and skin graftings
C. Multiple 'Z' plasty
D. Fat grafts

300. **Commonest indication for surgery in pectus excavatum is :**
A. Recurrent respiratory infections
B. Respiratory deficiency
C. Cosmetic reasons
D. Presses great vessels

301. **Absent clavicles are seen in :**
A. Cliedoacromial diastasis
B. Achondroplasia
C. Morquio disease
D. Oliver's disease

302. **Aberrant lamina dura is a feature of :**
A. Osteomalacia
B. Senile osteoporosis
C. Marfan's syndrome
D. Primary hyperparathyroidism

303. **Most common cause of genu valgum in India is :**
A. Trauma
B. Rickets
C. Scurvy
D. Fluorosis

304. **Cobb's angle is measured by :**
A. Kyphosis
B. Scoliosis
C. Lordosis
D. Lateral flexion

305. **Bilateral CDH (Congenital Dislocation of Hip) shows all, except :**
A. Waddling gait
B. Trendelenburg positive
C. Distorted Shelton's lin
D. Lordosis
E. Deep acetabulum

Ans. 298. C 299. B 300. C 301. A 302. C 303. B
304. B 305. E

306. **Pectus carinatum is seen in :**
A. Cretinism
B. Senile osteoporosis
C. Osteogenesis imperfecta
D. Chronic asthma

307. **Calcaneal deformity is most commonly due to :**
A. Malunited calcaneum
B. Ruptured tend calcaneus
C. Lateral peroneal nerve injury
D. Atrophy of gastrosoleus

308. **In which of the following syndrome is polydactyly common :**
A. Ellis-van Creveld syndrome
B. Tar syndrome
C. Fong syndrome
D. Rubinstein-Taybi syndrome

309. **Musculoskeletal abnormalities in neurofibromatosis is :**
A. Hypertrophy of limb B. Scoliosis
C. Pseudoarthrosis D. All of the above

310. **Dennis Brown splint is useful in :**
A. Genu valgum B. Genu varus
C. L.T.E. varus D. Fracture ulna

311. **Phocomelia is caused by ingestion of ——— during pregnancy.**
A. Steroids B. Tetracycline
C. Thalidomide D. Barbiturates

312. **Treatment of CTEV should begin :**
A. Soon after birth B. After discharge from hospital
C. After one month D. At 2 years

313. **Trident hand is seen in :**
A. Mucopolysaccharidosis B. Achondroplasia
C. Diaphyseal achalasia D. Chondrodysplasia

314. **Most important pathology in club foot is :**
A. Congenital talonavicular dislocation
B. Tightening of tendoachilles
C. Calcaneal fracture
D. Lateral derangement

Ans. 306. D 307. B 308. A 309. D 310. C 311. C
312. A 313. B 314. A

315. In congenital dislocation of hip, all of the following are true, except :
   A. Real shortening
   B. Telescoping +ve
   C. Trendelenburg test positive
   D. Head of femur is downwards
316. Pes Cavus is caused by :
   A. Weakness of intrinsic muscles of the foot
   B. Excessive tone of intrinsic muscles
   C. Collapse of the arch
   D. Fracture of calcaneum
317. Adventitious bursa is :
   A. Normal
   B. Abnormal over friction site
   C. An infected defect
   D. A congenital cyst
318. The clinical examination to differentiate compensatory scoliosis from structural scoliosis is :
   A. The patient is asked to sit down.
   B. The patient is asked to bend on both the sides one after the other.
   C. The patient is asked to extend the spine and try to look at the ceiling.
   D. The patient is asked to lean forward.
   E. Patient pelvis is held from behind and he asked to look at one side or the other.
319. In case of meningocele what other congenital deformity one should look for :
   A. Congenital dislocation of hip
   B. Talipes equinovarus
   C. Genu valgum
   D. Paraplegia
   E. Cleft lip
320. Arachnoidactyly is :
   A. Overdevelopment of bone or an extremity
   B. Concerned with infective condition of brain
   C. Maldevelopment of an anatomic part
   D. Disease of bone related to a defect

Ans. 315. D 316. A 317. B 318. A 319. B 320. A

321. **Genu varum is seen in :**
A. Syphilis
B. Epiphyseal dysplasia
C. Dietary deficiency
D. Physiologic at birth

322. **Osteogenesis imperfecta is :**
A. Autosomal Dominant (AD)
B. Autosomal Recessive (AR)
C. Both AD and AR
D. Sex linked dominant

323. **Which is not a feature of equinus deformity in polio :**
A. Paralysis of tibialis anterior muscles
B. Gravity plays a role
C. Contracted gastrocnemius
D. Denervation

324. **Most common cause of scoliosis is :**
A. Trauma
B. Congenital
C. Paralytic
D. Postural

325. **Which is not a feature of pseudochondroplasia :**
A. Short limbs in comparison to trunk
B. Kyphosis
C. Normal size skull
D. None of the above

326. **Ollier's disease is found in :**
A. Metacarpal bones
B. Fibula
C. Tibia
D. Femur

327. **Which of the following is known as Legg-Calve's Perthe's disease :**
A. Osteochondritis of proximal femoral epiphysis
B. Slipped capital femoral epiphysis
C. Tuberculosis of hip
D. Septic arthritis of hip

328. **Deafness in cases of Paget's disease is due to :**
A. Thickened cranium
B. Narrowing of foramina of skull
C. Brain compression
D. Otosclerosis
E. None of the above

Ans. 321. B 322. C 323. C 324. D 325. D 326. A
327. A 328. D

329. Which of the following is not a feature of coxa-vara :
A. Increased external rotation of affected hip
B. Prominent greater trochanter of affected hip
C. +ve Trendelenburg sign
D. Lengthening of the affected limb

330. Spinal dysraphism includes following, except :
A. Meningocele
B. Diastematomyelia
C. Intraspinal lipoma
D. Lateral thoracic meningocele

331. The radiological findings in a case of Perthe's disease include all of the following, except :
A. Coxa magna
B. Flattening of capital femoral epiphysis
C. Irregular epiphyseal line
D. Reduction in joint space

332. Nail patella syndrome is mostly associated with :
A. Deformity of tibia
B. Deformity of skull
C. Irregular dentition
D. Deformity of pelvis
E. None of the above

333. Osteogenesis imperfecta is basically due to :
A. Calcium deficiency
B. Phosphorus deficiency
C. Failure to produce mature collagen fibres
D. Defective chondroblasts

334. Radiological evidence of spondylolisthesis includes :
A. Defect in pars interarticularis
B. Forward slip of the body of one vertebra upon another
C. Both of the above
D. None of the above

335. Which of the following muscles is/are found congenitally absent more frequently :
A. Sternocleidomastoid
B. Trapezius
C. Quadratus femoris
D. Serratus anterior

Ans. 329. D 330. A 331. D 332. D 333. C 334. C
335. B

336. Vertebra plana is caused by :

A. Malignancy B. Tuberculosis
C. Syphilis D. Eosinophilic granuloma

337. A child with blue sclera and multiple fractures has :

A. Rickets
B. Scurvy
C. Osteogenesis imperfecta
D. Achondroplasia

338. Cleidocranial dysostosis may show :

A. Wide foramen magnum B. Absence of clavicles
C. Coxa vara D. All of the above

339. Achondroplasia occurs as :

A. Autosomal recessive
B. Autosomal dominant
C. Sporadic new mutations
D. None of the above

340. Lambrinudi fusion is done for :

A. Paralytic pes calcaneus
B. Foot drop
C. Club foot
D. Flat foot

341. Regarding multiple exostosis, which of the following is untrue :

A. Familial disorder
B. Commonly occur in males
C. Develop in epiphysis of bone
D. May cause pressure symptoms

342. Brachycephaly occurs due to premature closure of ________ sutures.

A. Coronal B. Sagittal
C. Lambdoidal D. Parietal

343. Flat foot is most commonly seen in :

A. Toddlers
B. Os calcis fracture
C. Congenital vertical talus
D. Spastic peroneal muscles

Ans. **336. D** **337. C** **338. D** **339. C** **340. B** **341. C**
342. A **343. A**

344. **Congenital pseudoarthrosis of the tibia is probably :**
A. A developmental abnormality
B. Associated with neurofibromatosis
C. Due to an ununited intra-uterine fracture
D. Due to all of the above

345. **The word talipes refers to :**
A. Long feet with spidery toes
B. Club feet
C. Flat feet
D. Hammer toes

346. **Bone dysplasia is due to :**
A. Faulty nutrition
B. Faulty development
C. Parathyroid tumour
D. Trauma

347. **Idiopathic scoliosis is a :**
A. Lateral curvature of the spine
B. Rotation of the spine
C. Lateral curvature with rotation of the spine
D. Flexion deformity of the spine

348. **Metatarsus primus varus is a cause of :**
A. Pes cavus
B. Talipes equinovarus
C. Hallux varus
D. Hallux valgus

349. **Hammer toes :**
A. Do not develop adventitious bursa.
B. Are due to injury caused by a heavy object (e.g. a hammer) falling on the toes.
C. Is a type of Dupuytren's disease.
D. Can be relieved by supplying insoles.

350. **Not seen in flurosis :**
A. Osteoporosis
B. Calcification of ligaments & tendons
C. Mottling of teeth
D. None of the above

351. **Cartilage hair hypoplasia, false is :**
A. Short limb dwarfism
B. Sparse hair on trunk
C. T-cell dysfunction
D. Neutropenia

Ans. 344. D 345. B 346. B 347. C 348. D 349. C 350. A 351. D

352. **Ward's triangle is in response to :**
A. Congenital coxa vara
B. CDH
C. Torsion of femoral shaft
D. Neck of femur

353. **The characteristics of Morquio's disease include :**
A. Dwarfism
B. Subnormal/normal intelligence
C. Spinal kyphosis
D. Excessive excretion of kerato sulphate in urine
E. All of the above

354. **Main en triedent is :**
A. A small hand with flexed wrist.
B. Short and broad hand with fingers of equal length.
C. Long and narrow hand with long unequal fingers.
D. Relatively short hand with fused fingers.
E. Relatively broad hand with more than 5 fingers.

355. **Ectrodactylism is :**
A. Supernumerary digits
B. Overgrowth of fingers
C. Absence of digits
D. Webbing of fingers

356. **The level of the constricting nodule in case of a trigger finger is at :**
A. Neck of the corresponding metacarpal bone
B. Metacarpophalangeal joint
C. Proximal interphalangeal joint
D. Distal interphalangeal joint

357. **Mirror hand is :**
A. Reduplication of ulna
B. Congenital subluxation of ulna
C. Congenital subluxation of radius
D. Injury of hand with a broken piece of mirror
E. None of the above

Ans. 352. D 353. E 354. B 355. C 356. A 357. A

358. Recurrent dislocation of hip in meningomyelocele is because of :
A. Sciatic nerve palsy
B. Because of strong flexors and adductors
C. Congenital coxa vera
D. Limp musculature

359. In Humper's lump, adventitious bursa is commonest on :
A. C_5 B. C_6
C. C_7 D. T_1

360. In Valus deformity, defect lies in joint :
A. Calcaneocuboid B. Talocuboid
C. Talocalcaneal D. Talonavicular

361. Flexion-adduction deformity of hip is seen in :
A. Unreduced posterior dislocation of hip
B. Anterior dislocation of hip joint
C. Central dislocation of hip
D. Impacted intracapsular fracture of neck of femur

362. Which of the following is the commonest combination of deformities in 'club-foot' :
A. Equino-varus B. Equino-valgus
C. Calcaneovalgus D. Equino-cavovarus

363. Monostotic fibrous dysplasia is chiefly a disease of :
A. New born babies B. Children
C. Adolescents D. Adult males
E. Adult females

364. 'Gunstock' deformity occurs as a complication of which fracture:
A. Supracondylar fracture
B. Capitulum fracture
C. Fracture neck of radius
D. Fracture lateral epicondyle humerus

365. Congenital pseudoarthrosis is seen in :
A. Tibia-Fibula B. Femur
C. Femur-Tibia D. Hip joint

Ans. 358. B 359. C 360. D 361. A 362. A 363. C
364. A 365. A

366. True about Robert's pelvis is :
A. Triradiate inlet
B. Single sacral alamissing
C. Both sacral ala missing
D. None of the above

367. In a new born child, abduction and internal rotation produces a click sound. It is :
A. Otorolani's sign B. Telescoping sign
C. Mc Murray's sign D. Lachman's sign

368. Known factors for 'Idiopathic scoliosis' :
A. Unknown B. Polio
C. Postural D. Congenital

369. Treatment of club foot should begin :
A. As soon as possible after birth
B. 1 month after birth
C. 1 year after birth
D. None of the above

370. Most popular sign of hip dysplasia in new born is :
A. Trendelenburg sign B. Galazi's sign
C. Ortolani's sign D. Telescopic test

371. After closed reduction of congenital dislocation of hip the limb could be immobilised in :
A. Frog position B. Human position
C. Bachelor plaster D. Any of the above

372. Club foot seen in a 15 years old could be treated successfully by :
A. Appropriate foot wear B. Soft tissue operation
C. Triple arthrodesis D. Quadriple fusion

373. Regarding cervical rib, which of the following is true :
A. It is always bony in nature
B. It can always be felt
C. It always produces symptoms
D. Symptoms may include ischaemic muscle pain in forearm and trophic changes in fingers

---

Ans. 366. C 367. A 368. A 369. A 370. C 371. D
372. C 373. D

374. **Sprengel's deformity of scapula is :**
A. Undescended/elevated scapula
B. Undescended neck of scapula
C. Exostosis scapula
D. None of the above

375. **Fibrous dysplasia with pigmentation and sexual precocity is seen in :**
A. Albright's syndrome B. Neurofibromatosis
C. Turner's syndrome D. Klinefelter's syndrome

376. **Vertebra plana is seen in :**
A. Eosinophilic granuloma B. Multiple myeloma
C. Perthes disease D. Paget's disease

Match the following (Ques. 377 to 381) :

377. **Slipped capital femoral epiphysis** a) 0-5 years
378. **Osteo-arthritis :** b) 5-10 years
379. **Tubercular arthritis :** c) 10-15 years
380. **Perthe's disease :** d) Above 4 years
381. **Congenital dislocation of hip:** e) Any age

382. **Club foot is when :**
A. Plantar flexion
B. Plantar flexion with inversion
C. Plantar flexion with eversion
D. Plantar extension

383. **Which is not true in mandibular facial dystosis :**
A. Ocular defect B. Microtia
C. Webbing of neck D. Mandibular hypoplasia

384. **Which is not a heritable collagen disorder :**
A. Homocystinuria B. Ehlers Danlos syndrome
C. Marfan's syndrome D. Down's syndrome

385. **In multiple exostosis, most common age of presentation is :**
A. 2—10 B. 16—25
C. 35—45 D. Above 60

386. **Hallux valgus is often associated with :**
A. Hallux rigidus B. Bunion
C. Gout D. Fracture tibia

Ans. 374. A 375. A 376. A 377. C 378. D 379. E
380. B 381. A 382. B 383. C 384. A 385. A
386. B

387. **Congenital dislocation of knock knee causes ——— deformity.**
A. Varus B. Valgus
C. Hyperextensions D. Flexion

388. **Most common cause of kyphosis in a male is :**
A. Congenital B. TB
C. Trauma D. Secondaries

389. **Cattrell's classification is useful for :**
A. CDH B. CTEV
C. Perthes' disease D. Fracture neck femur

390. **Tendons involved in de Quervain's synovitis :**
A. Extensor carpi longus and abductor pollicis brevis (APB).
B. Extensor carpi longus & abductor pollicis longus.
C. Extensor pollicis brevis & abductor pollicis longus.
D. Extensor carpi ulnaris & abductor pollicis brevis.

391. **Which one of the following statements regarding open spina bifida is incorrect:**
A. It is a neural tube defect.
B. It may be associated with raised amniotic fluid alpha-fetoproteins.
C. Affected parents have five per cent chance of having affected child.
D. 75% will survive even in the absence of surgical treatment.

392. **Flexible flat foot is seen in all, except :**
A. Physiological B. Elderly
C. Vertical talus D. Hypermobility

393. **Phacomelia is :**
A. Complete absence of extremities
B. Partial absence of extremities
C. Absence of long bones
D. Absence of short bones

394. **Club foot is ——— defect.**
A. Congenital B. Intrinsic muscles of foot
C. Birth injury D. Acquired

395. **Sclerosis of vertebral end plates can occur in following, except :**
A. Sarcoidosis B. Osteoporosis
C. Rheumatoid arthritis D. Healing osteomalacia

Ans. 387. B 388. B 389. C 390. C 391. D 392. C
393. C 394. B 395. B

396. **In correction of clubfoot by manipulation, which deformity should be corrected first :**
A. Forefoot adduction
B. Varus
C. Equinus
D. Internal tibial torsion

397. **Tendon transfer in polio is done at the age of :**
A. Less than 6 months
B. 6 months to 1 year
C. 2 years
D. 5 years

398. **Earliest changes in Perthes' disease is seen by :**
A. X-ray
B. CT
C. MRI
D. US
E. Nuclear scan

399. **Accessory navicular is called :**
A. Os trigonum
B. Os tibiale internum
C. Os tibiale externum
D. Os navicular

400. **Dysplasia epiphysis hemimelia is :**
A. Trevor's disease
B. Blount's disease
C. Streeter's dysplasia
D. Leri's disease

401. **Triradiate pelvis is seen in :**
A. Osteomalacia
B. Senile osteoporosis
C. Paget's disease
D. Hypothyroidism

402. **Which of the defect in talipes equinovarus is corrected last :**
A. Adduction of fore foot
B. Equinus deformity
C. Rotation at ankle
D. All together

403. **A neonate has an assymetric Moro's reflex, social smile is normal. On examination weak or absent abduction of shoulder and supination of forearm. The lesion lies at :**
A. C_{3-6}
B. C_{3-4}
C. C_{7-8}
D. T_{1-4}

404. **Which of the following is true regarding aneurysmal bone cyst :**
A. Characteristically elliptical in long bones.
B. More common after the age of 50 yrs.
C. More common is vertebra
D. Due to atherosclerosis

Ans. 396. A 397. D 398. E 399. C 400. A 401. A
402. B 403. C 404. A

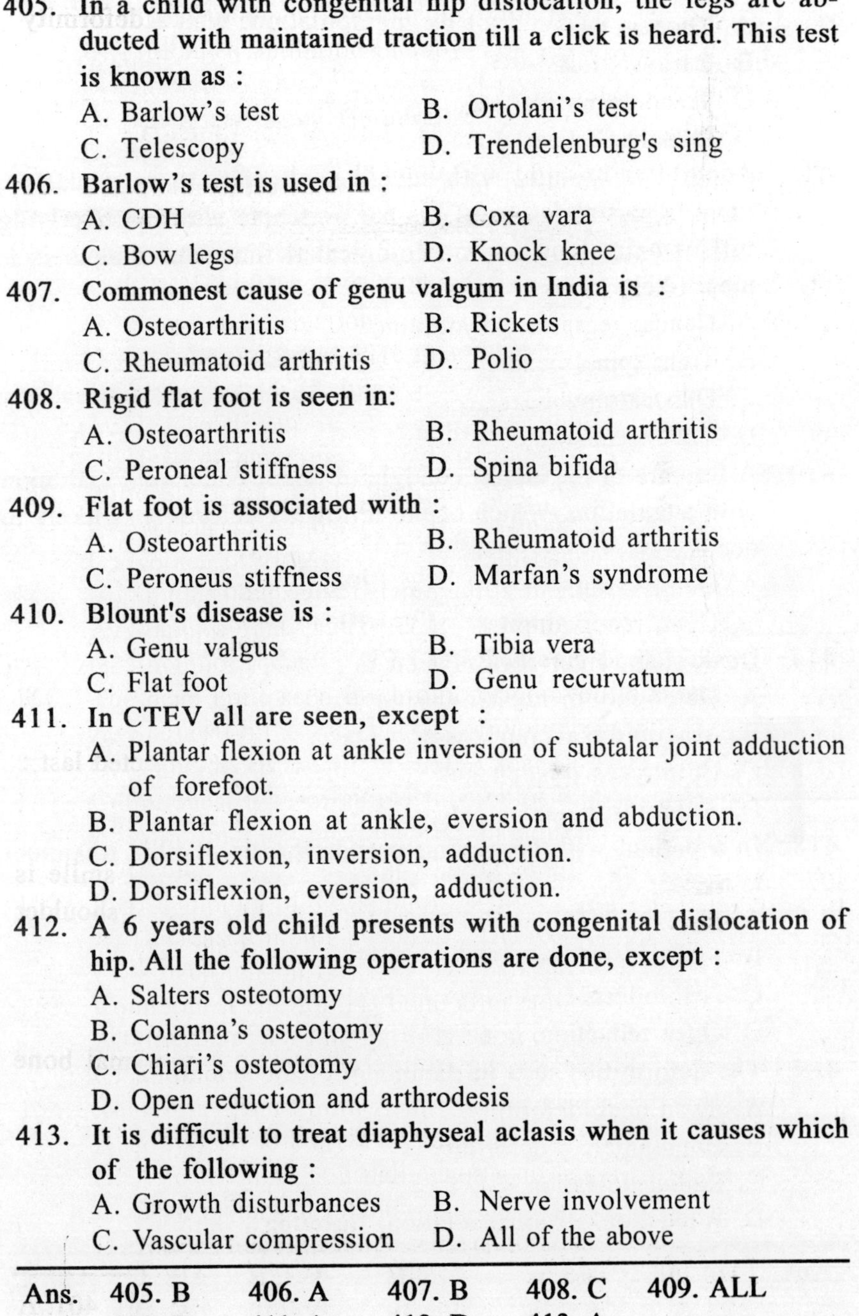

405. **In a child with congenital hip dislocation, the legs are abducted with maintained traction till a click is heard. This test is known as :**
A. Barlow's test B. Ortolani's test
C. Telescopy D. Trendelenburg's sing

406. **Barlow's test is used in :**
A. CDH B. Coxa vara
C. Bow legs D. Knock knee

407. **Commonest cause of genu valgum in India is :**
A. Osteoarthritis B. Rickets
C. Rheumatoid arthritis D. Polio

408. **Rigid flat foot is seen in:**
A. Osteoarthritis B. Rheumatoid arthritis
C. Peroneal stiffness D. Spina bifida

409. **Flat foot is associated with :**
A. Osteoarthritis B. Rheumatoid arthritis
C. Peroneus stiffness D. Marfan's syndrome

410. **Blount's disease is :**
A. Genu valgus B. Tibia vera
C. Flat foot D. Genu recurvatum

411. **In CTEV all are seen, except :**
A. Plantar flexion at ankle inversion of subtalar joint adduction of forefoot.
B. Plantar flexion at ankle, eversion and abduction.
C. Dorsiflexion, inversion, adduction.
D. Dorsiflexion, eversion, adduction.

412. **A 6 years old child presents with congenital dislocation of hip. All the following operations are done, except :**
A. Salters osteotomy
B. Colanna's osteotomy
C. Chiari's osteotomy
D. Open reduction and arthrodesis

413. **It is difficult to treat diaphyseal aclasis when it causes which of the following :**
A. Growth disturbances B. Nerve involvement
C. Vascular compression D. All of the above

Ans. 405. B 406. A 407. B 408. C 409. ALL
410. B 411. A 412. D 413. A

414. The fixed flexion deformity of hip can be tested by :
A. Thomas test
B. Barlow's test
C. Trendelenburg's test
D. Lachman's test

415. A child is brought with severe scoliosis. On examination, there is partial fusion of lumbar vertebrae with an overlying tuft of hair along and neurological deficit. The diagnosis is most likely to be :
A. Caudal regression syndrome
B. Tight spinal band
C. Diasteatomyelia
D. Coccygeal cyst

416. A fracture of the lateral condyle of femur underwent malunion with angulation. Which of the following deformity is likely to occur :
A. Genu varum B. Genu valgum
C. Genu recurvatum D. Tibia vara

417. Beak shaped vertebra is seen in :
A. Osteochondrodystrophy
B. Mucopolysaccharidosis
C. Epiphyses dysgenesis
D. Achondroplasia

418. In a patient with congenital pseudarthrosis of tibia treatment is by :
A. Excision
B. Fibular grafting
C. Arthrodesis
D. Open reduction, bone grafting and internal fixation

419. The deformities seen in rheumatoid hand are all except :
A. Swan neck deformity
B. Boutonniere's deformity
C. Radial deviation
D. Adduction, external rotation, flexation

Ans. 414. A 415. C 416. B 417. B 418. C 419. C

420. **All the statements regarding congenital radio ulnar syntosis are true, except :**
A. Fusion of both ends of the radius and ulnar
B. Fixed in mid prone position
C. Pulled elbow is a differential diagnosis
D. Even with operative treatment prognosis is guarded

421. **The level of amputation is best indicated by :**
A. Age of the patient B. Venous pulsation
C. Doppler D. Cyanosis

422. **In Vokman's ischaemic contracture, prevention is done by :**
A. Elevation
B. Padded plaster + elevation
C. Splitting of cast
D. Tight plaster

423. **Hyoid bone is removed in :**
A. Carotid body tumour B. Thyroid adenoma
C. Thyroglossal cyst D. Medium thyroidectomy

424. **Genslen's operation is for :**
A. Sacroiliac subluxation
B. Recurrent shoulder dislocation
C. Cervical spondylosis
D. T.B. arthritis of knee joint

425. **The Risser turnbuckle cast is used to :**
A. Correct deformity occurring in the union of a fracture
B. Correct kyphosis
C. Overcome fixed flexion of the hip joint
D. Correct scoliosis

426. **Arthrodesis of the following is done to correct flat foot, except :**
A. Cervical spine B. Upper thoracic spine
C. Lower thoracic spine D. Lumbar spine

427. **von Rosen splint is used in the treatment of :**
A. Clubfoot
B. Congenital coxa vera
C. Congenital dislocation
D. Leg Calve Perthes disease

Ans. 420. A 421. C 422. C 423. C 424. A 425. D
426. D 427. C

428. **Installation treatment in osteomyelitis is :**
   A. Continuous suction + continuous drainage
   B. Intermittent suction + continuous drainage
   C. Continuous suction + intermittent drainage
   D. Intermittent suction + intermittent drainage

429. **Factors required in bone transplantation include following, except :**
   A. Osteogenecity of bone cells
   B. Surviving bone graft cells
   C. Induction
   D. Immune response
   E. Alkaline phosphatase inhibitors

430. **The preferred site for aspiration of knee is :**
   A. Through the middle of ligamentum patella
   B. Just above the patella in the middle
   C. Just above and medial to patella
   D. Just above and lateral to patella

431. **In adult patients requiring bilateral hip surgery the aetiological process in the majority of cases would be expected to be :**
   A. Avascular necrosis
   B. Degenerative joint disease
   C. Congenital dysplasias
   D. Residual septic arthritis

432. **The antibiotic of choice in actinomycotic osteomyelitis is :**
   A. Chloramphenicol   B. Penicillin
   C. Nystatin   D. Sulphadiazine

433. **Which of the following is critical area of pulleys :**
   A. Area between wrist and distal palmer crease.
   B. Area from distal palmer crease to proximal interphalangeal joint.
   C. Area from distal interphalangeal joint upto tip of the finger.
   D. None of the above.

Ans. 428. B   429. E   430. D   431. B   432. B   433. B

434. **During the surgical procedure :**
A. Tendons should be repaired before nerves
B. Nerves should be repaired before tendons
C. Tendons should not be repaired at the same time
D. None is true

435. **Symes amputation is for :**
A. Lower end of femur
B. Lower end of tibia
C. Lower end of tibia + fibula
D. Lower end of radius + ulnar

436. **Camer wire is a :**
A. Ligature B. Stitch
C. Splint D. Cast

437. **Repeated closed reduction in hip joint is :**
A. Rewarding
B. Less damaging than surgical
C. Contraindicated
D. Unsuccessful

438. **Calcaneus lengthening is done in :**
A. Equinus deformity B. Cuboid deformity
C. Flat foot D. Foot drop

439. **Gallow's splint is used for children below——— years age.**
A. 2 B. 5
C. 9 D. 12

440. **A plaster of Paris splint used to immobilise a fracture should :**
A. Immobilise the joints above and below the fracture.
B. Not immobilise any joint below the fracture.
C. Be applied dry and then sprayed with water.
D. Always be put on and left for 48 hours completely surrounding the affecting limb.

441. **Distance from the tip of greater trochanter in thigh amputation is ——— inches.**
A. 5 B. 7
C. 9 D. 11

Ans. 434. A 435. C 436. C 437. D438. A 439. A
440. A 441. D

442. **Meyer's operation is done for :**
A. Dislocation of patella B. Fracture neck of femur
C. Dislocation of shoulder D. Fracture fibula

443. **Intervertebral disc prolapse is treated chemically by :**
A. Hyalase B. Chymotrypsin
C. Chymopapain D. Elastase

444. **Chemical synovectomy is done by :**
A. Osmic acid B. Chymopapain
C. Chymotrypsin D. Trypsin

445. **Non-dynamic splint is :**
A. Banjo B. Opponens
C. Cock-up D. Brand

446. **One of the following is not the eponym associated with the operation for ingrowing toe nail :**
A. Quenu B. Zadik
C. Fowler D. Girdlestone

447. **A Gigli saw is :**
A. An electrically driven circular bone saw
B. A pneumatically driven bone saw
C. A short straight bone saw
D. A long twisted wire bone saw

448. **The anterior operative approach in diseased knee is most suitable for :**
A. Synovectomy
B. Excision menisci
C. Repair of collateral ligaments
D. Arthrodesis

449. **Regarding McMurry's osteotomy :**
A. It is done for certain fracture of neck femur.
B. Adduction type of fracture is converted into abduction type of fracture.
C. A hip spica/internal fixation plate is applied for stability of fragments.
D. All the above are true.

Ans. 442. B 443. C 444. A 445. C 446. D 447. D
448. D 449. D

450. Charnley's principles of total hip replacement comprises of :
A. Thick elastic socker (Acetabular cup) of HDP i.e. high density polyethylene.
B. Femoral head of (stainless steel) small diameter.
C. Shifting of greater trochanter more laterally.
D. Displacement of fulcrum medially.
E. All of the above.

451. Self-curing acrylic cement is :
A. Polymerized methylmethacrylate + peroxide activator.
B. Methylmethacrylate monomer + Tertiary amine initiator.
C. A product made from combination of A and B.
D. None of the above.

452. Indications for arthrodesis in knee are all the following except :
A. Osteoarthritis (very advance stage).
B. Old comminuted painful intra-articular fractures.
C. Tuberculosis knee with marked damage to articular surfaces.
D. Marked degree of flexion contracture of knee.

453. Pointing index finger during clasping is a sign of :
A. Radial nerve injury
B. Median nerve injury
C. Ulnar nerve injury
D. Circumflex humeral nerve injury
E. Posterior interosseous nerve injury

454. The poorest results (recover) are noticed in the repair of injured:
A. Ulnar nerve
B. Median nerve
C. Sciatic nerve
D. Posterior tibial nerve

455. After repair of an injured peripheral nerve the estimated rate of functional recovery per month is :
A. 1/2"
B. 1"
C. 1.5"
D. 2"

456. The continuing pain after a peripheral nerve injury repair can be overcome by :
A. P.O.P. cost
B. Narcotics
C. Passive and active motions of the affected limb
D. None of the above

Ans. 450. E 451. C 452. D 453. B 454. C 455. B 456. C

457. **Treatment of acute pain in gout, is except :**
A. Phenylbutazone B. Codeine
C. Allopuriano D. Prednisolone

458. **Osteotomy is best indicated in :**
A. Spondylolisthesis B. Cervical spondylitis
C. Lumbar disc prolapse D. Ankylosing spondylosis

459. **Amputated limb is preserved in :**
A. Dry cold B. Cold saline
C. Ringer lactate D. At room temperature

460. **Frost bite of a limb is best treated by :**
A. Graduated warming B. Rapid warming
C. Amputation D. Lumbar sympathectomy

461. **Amputation is not indicated in :**
A. Maduromycosis B. Chronic osteomyelitis
C. Buerger's disease D. Gas gangrene

462. **Lumbar spiral osteotomy is indicated in :**
A. Spondylolisthesis
B. Tuberculosis of the spine
C. Lumbar canal paresis
D. Ankylosing spondylosis

463. **Triple fusion of joint is done at :**
A. Ankle B. Subtalar joint
C. Calcaneocuboid D. Talocalcaneal

464. **Radioactive dye used in bone scan is :**
A. 99 m Tc B. I^{131}
C. Strontium 99 D. Gallium

465. **Best bone graft is :**
A. Allograft B. Autograft
C. Deproteinised graft D. Demineralised graft

466. **Hemi exposure of the femur goes through :**
A. Vastus medialis B. Vastus lateralis
C. Vastus intermedius D. Rectus femoris

467. **Bone graft with maximum osteogenic potential is :**
A. Fresh autograft B. Fresh cortical autograft
C. Osteoperiosteal graft D. Vascular bone graft

Ans. 457. C 458. D 459. A 460. A 461. B 462. D
463. B 464. A 465. D 466. D 467. D

468. **Phemister bone graft principle is :**
A. To stimulate osteogenesis by freshing bone ends.
B. Stimulate osteogenesis by multiple drilling at site of non-union.
C. To stimulate osteogenesis by stripping the periosteum.
D. To add bone graft without disturbing site of non-union.

469. **The most popular tendon transfer for foot drop in leprosy is :**
A. Tibialis anterior laterally
B. Peroneus longus to the dorsum
C. Tibialis posterior to the dorsum
D. Extensor hallucis longus to the metatarsal neck

470. **Operative procedure of choice in Pott's paraplegia is :**
A. Laminectomy
B. Costotransversectomy
C. Spinal fusion
D. Anteriolateral decompression

471. **Bone grafting is recommended to repair the :**
A. Proximal 2/3 of fibula B. Lateral end of clavicle
C. Lower end of ulna D. Lower end of radius
E. Patella

472. **Osteoclasis can be used to :**
A. Correct deformity of the tibia due to rickets
B. Curette an osteoclastoma
C. Correct deformity due to Paget's disease
D. Correct a ricketed rosary

473. **Local application of the following drug is used for eradication of pseudomonas infection from the wound :**
A. Acriflavin solution B. Eusol paraffin
C. Acetic acid D. Tincture Iodine

474. **Bone scan imaging with Tc-99m phosphate, if performed within 72 hours, can predict avascular necrosis with :**
A. 90% accuracy B. 80% accuracy
C. 75% accuracy D. 50% accuracy

Ans. 468. A 469. D 470. D 471. D 472. A 473. C
474. A

475. **A plaster of Paris spica is :**
A. A metal footpiece incorporated in the plaster for weight bearing.
B. A plaster bandage used for avulsion fractures of the terminal phalanx of a finger.
C. A plaster bandage around the pelvis and upper thigh with a resulting pattern that resembles an ear of wheat.
D. A metal pin which is used for traction purposes of a plaster cast.

476. **The preferred treatment for unicameral bone cyst is :**
A. X-ray therapy
B. Surgical exposure and collapse of cavity
C. Surgical curettage and bone graft
D. Create a fracture and allow to heal

477. **Macewon's osteotomy is performed in cases of :**
A. Coxa vara B. Tibia vara
C. Genu valgum D. Tom Smith disease

478. **Which one of the following operations is inappropriate in the treatment of osteoarthrosis :**
A. Synovectomy B. Arthrodesis
C. Arthroplasty D. Osteotomy

479. **SP nailing is indicated in :**
A. Fresh fracture with comminution
B. Fresh fracture in adults
C. Fresh fracture in children
D. Old fracture with comminution
E. Fracture wrist

480. **The effect of excision of radial head in children is :**
A. Varus deformity B. Valgus deformity
C. Lengthening of limb D. Restriction of supination
E. All of the above

481. **Operative indications for paraplegia is :**
A. Progressive motor loss inspite of conservative movement.
B. Loss of consciousness.
C. Non-improvement of sensory loss within 1 week.
D. Non-improvement of motor loss within 3 weeks.
E. Incontinence of urine.

Ans. 475. C 476. C 477. D 478. A 479. B 480. B
481. A

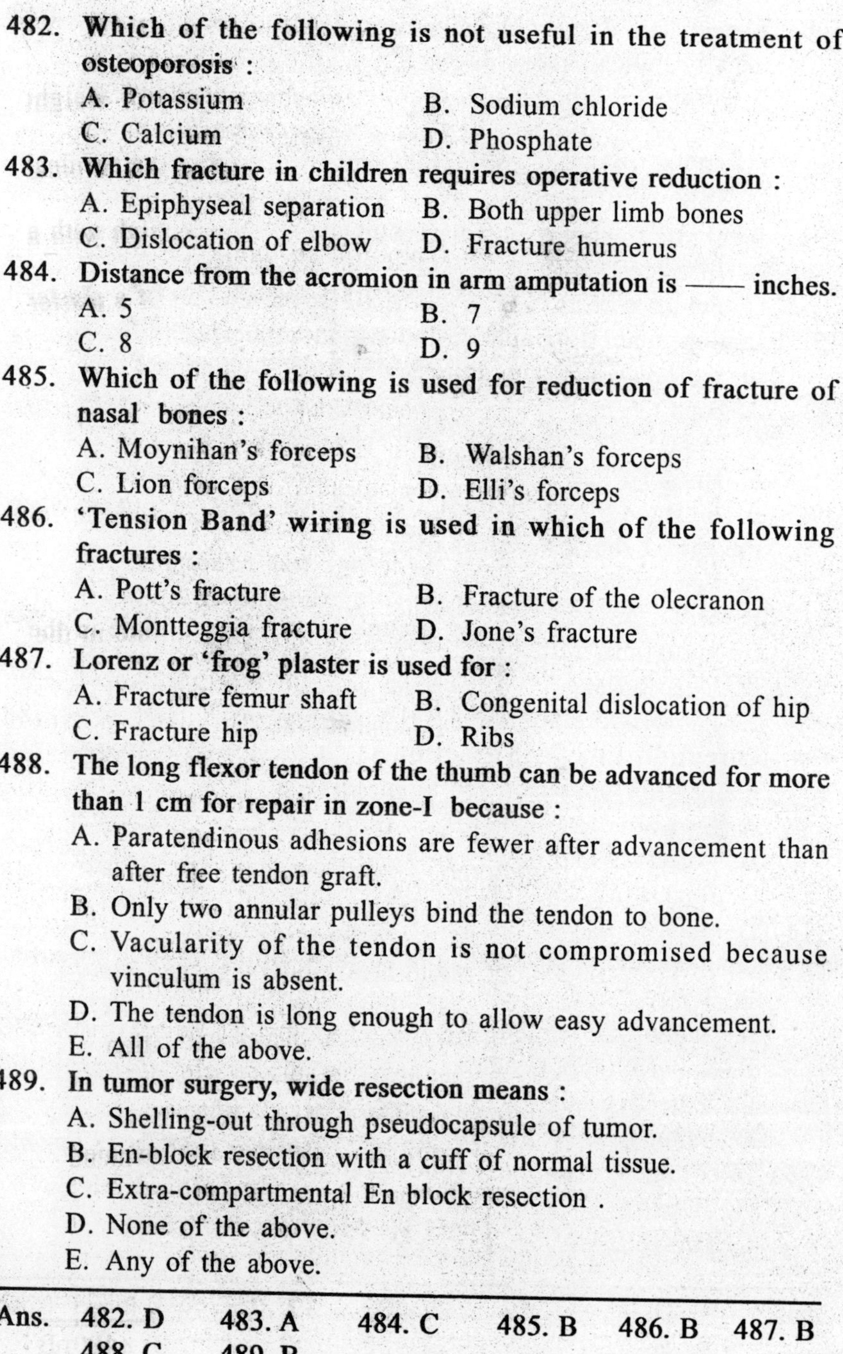

482. **Which of the following is not useful in the treatment of osteoporosis :**
A. Potassium B. Sodium chloride
C. Calcium D. Phosphate

483. **Which fracture in children requires operative reduction :**
A. Epiphyseal separation B. Both upper limb bones
C. Dislocation of elbow D. Fracture humerus

484. **Distance from the acromion in arm amputation is —— inches.**
A. 5 B. 7
C. 8 D. 9

485. **Which of the following is used for reduction of fracture of nasal bones :**
A. Moynihan's forceps B. Walshan's forceps
C. Lion forceps D. Elli's forceps

486. **'Tension Band' wiring is used in which of the following fractures :**
A. Pott's fracture B. Fracture of the olecranon
C. Montteggia fracture D. Jone's fracture

487. **Lorenz or 'frog' plaster is used for :**
A. Fracture femur shaft B. Congenital dislocation of hip
C. Fracture hip D. Ribs

488. **The long flexor tendon of the thumb can be advanced for more than 1 cm for repair in zone-I because :**
A. Paratendinous adhesions are fewer after advancement than after free tendon graft.
B. Only two annular pulleys bind the tendon to bone.
C. Vacularity of the tendon is not compromised because vinculum is absent.
D. The tendon is long enough to allow easy advancement.
E. All of the above.

489. **In tumor surgery, wide resection means :**
A. Shelling-out through pseudocapsule of tumor.
B. En-block resection with a cuff of normal tissue.
C. Extra-compartmental En block resection .
D. None of the above.
E. Any of the above.

Ans. 482. D 483. A 484. C 485. B 486. B 487. B
488. C 489. B

490. A persistent drop of blood pressure in an acutely injured patient usually indicates loss of :
A. 500 cc of blood
B. 500 cc of plasma
C. 500 cc of extracellular fluid
D. 1500 cc of blood

491. Ideal site for bone graft harvesting is :
A. Iliac crest
B. Skull bones
C. Femur cortex
D. Tibial cortex

492. In flap method of amputation which structure is kept shorter than the level of amputation :
A. Skin
B. Muscles
C. Vessels
D. Nerves
E. Bone

493. In the stage of spinal shock what is lost which reappears when the spinal shock becomes over :
A. Sensory loss
B. Motor power
C. Superficial reflexes
D. Deep reflexes
E. Paraplegic bladder

494. Direction in which traction is to be applied to reduce a dislocation temporomandibular joint is :
A. Forwards and upwards
B. Forwards and downwards
C. Backwards and downwards
D. Backwards and upwards

495. Open reductional internal fixation is almost always essential in :
A. Salter type-I fracture
B. Salter type-II fracture
C. Salter type-III fracture
D. Salter type-IV fracture

496. In collagen, drug most concentrated is :
A. Heparin
B. Chloroquine
C. Griseofulvin
D. Colchicine

Ans. 490. D 491. A 492. D 493. D 494. B 495. D 496. D

497. Management in case of rupture of disc at L_5S_1 is :
A. Emergency removal
B. Joint fusion
C. Immobilization for 2 weeks with spinal back
D. Traction

498. Points of importance in bone transplantation, are all, except:
A. Osteogenic activity of graft
B. Great survival
C. Induction
D. Increased alkaline phosphatase inhibitors

499. Commonest defect arising due to hip prosthesis :
A. Neck and shaft angle more
B. More anteversion
C. Inadequate excision of neck of femur
D. More retroversion

500. The maximum weight that can be used in skin traction is :
A. 6 Kg B. 4 Kg
C. 10 Kg D. 12 Kg

501. Treatment of a bone cyst with excision and bone chips grafting results in :
A. No chance of recurrence
B. Remote chance of recurrence
C. 2-3% recurrence
D. 5-10% recurrence

502. All the following require operative reduction, except :
A. Patella
B. Olecranon
C. Condyle of humerus
D. Outer 1/3rd of radius

503. In hand injuries, first to be repaired is :
A. Bone
B. Tendon
C. Skin
D. Nerve

Ans. **497. C** **498. D** **499. A** **500. B** **501. B** **502. C** **503. C**

504. **A man cuts himself across the palm of the right hand over the distal palmar crease three hours before presenting himself at the casualty. On examination he is unable to flex the middle and distal joints of the ring finger. Extension is normal. There is no sensory loss. Besides antibiotics and antitetanus globulin, the most appropriate treatment for the patient would be :**
A. Primary suture of flexor digitorum sublimis and flexor digitorum profundus tendons.
B. Primary repair of flexor digitorum profundus and excision of flexor digitorum sublimis.
C. Secondary repair of flexor digitorum profundus and excision of flexor digitorum sublimis.
D. Secondary excision of both tendons and great to replace flexor digitorum profundus.

505. **One of the following is regarded as the best prosthesis :**
A. Suction socket prosthesis
B. Syme prosthesis
C. Patellar tendon involved prosthesis
D. None of the above

506. **Gritti Stokes amputation is :**
A. Amputation through knee
B. Transcondylar amputation
C. Below knee amputation
D. None of the above

507. **For Lobster hand, treatment includes :**
A. No treatment
B. Orthotic device
C. Reconstructive surgery
D. Tendon transplantation

508. **Best revolutionised prosthesis for knee surgery :**
A. Suction B. Symes
C. Canadian D. Patellar tendon

509. **McMurray's osteotomy is based on the following principle :**
A. Biological B. Mechanical
C. Bio-mechanical D. Bio-technical

Ans. **504. B** **505. A** **506. B** **507. C** **508. A** **509. C**

510. **Which of the following may have malignant degeneration following radiotherapy :**
A. Giant cell tumor B. Bone cyst
C. Fibrous dysplasia D. Chondroblastoma
E. All of the above

511. **Which of the following muscles can not be expected to undergo phasic conversion with transfer and physiotherapy :**
A. Peroneus longus B. Peroneus brevis
C. Tibialis anterior D. Tibialis posterior
E. Hamstring muscles

512. **Irradiation causes :**
A. Paget's disease of breast B. Paget's disease of skin
C. Ewing's tumour D. Osteosarcoma

513. **Calcium content of bone is increased by :**
A. Prolonged immobilization
B. Hyperparathyroidism
C. Corticosteroids
D. Oestrogen

514. **Short wave diathermy is used for all of the following, except:**
A. Back pain B. Hemophilic joint
C. Osteoarthrosis D. None of the above

515. **At the present time total hip replacements using methylmethocrylate are limited to patients over the age of :**
A. 35 B. 45
C. 55 D. 65
E. 70

516. **Stump pain is releaved by :**
A. Continuous tapping on the stump
B. Lowering-up the stump
C. Using steroids
D. Using analgesics

517. **An ideal stump should have all, except :**
A. Skin without tension over the stump.
B. Opposite group of muscles sutured over the bone.
C. Skin firmly attached to subcutaneous tissue.
D. Full range of movements at the joint proximal to the site of amputation.

Ans. 510. E 511. A 512. D 513. D 514. B 515. D
516. A 517. C

518. **Osteoclasis can be used to :**
   A. Correct deformity of the tibia due to rickets
   B. Curette an osteoclastoma
   C. Correct deformity due to Paget's disease
   D. Correct a ricketed rosary

Match the following (Quest. 519 to 524) :

	Joint	*Appropriate position for arthrodesis*
519.	**Shoulder**	A. Full extension
520.	**Elbow**	B. Right Angle (Neutral position)
521.	**Wrist**	C. Full extension
522.	**Hip**	D. 50° abduction, 20° flexion, and 20° internal rotation
523.	**Knee**	E. 90°
524.	**Ankle**	F. 10°-20° extension

525. **In hand surgery which area is called 'No man's land':**
   A. Proximal phalanx
   B. Distal phalanx
   C. Between distal palmer crease and proximal phalanx
   D. Wrist

526. **Which of the following statements about Pulsating Magnetic Field Therapy (PMFT) is not true :**
   A. A magnetic field of extremely low frequency and ultra low intensity is effective.
   B. It is different from magnetic therapy.
   C. PMFT is useful in the treatment of osteoarthritis.
   D. It is also useful in promoting callus formation.
   E. It is not useful in the relief of pain in the musculoskeletal system.

527. **Total hip replacement is done in all, except :**
   A. Septic arthritis
   B. Inflammatory arthritis
   C. Osteoarthritis
   D. Osteonecrosis femur head

Ans. 518. A 519. D 520. E 521. F 522. A 523. C
524. B 525. C 526. E 527. A

528. **Faradic foot bath is used in :**
A. Paraplegia B. Foot drop
C. Quadriplegia D. All of the above

529. **Aeroplane splint is used in :**
A. Fracture displacement to elbow
B. Brachial plexus injury
C. Cervical spine injury
D. Scoliosis

530. **Level of amputation is best indicated by :**
A. Age of patient B. Venous pulsation
C. Doppler D. Cyanosis

531. **Which of the following is used in osteoporosis for decreasing bone resorption and increasing bone formation :**
A. Teriparatide B. Calcitonin
C. Strontium ranelate D. Bisphosphonate

532. **Not a treatment for chronic backache :**
A. NSAID
B. Bed rest for months
C. Exercises
D. Epidural steroid injection

533. **Myodesis is contraindicated in :**
A. Children B. Tumor
C. Ischemia D. Paralysis

534. **High tibial osteotomy are all true except :**
A. Not > 30 degree correction can be achieved
B. Done through cancellous bone
C. High chance of recurrence
D. It is done unicompartmental OA

535. **Emergency treatment of acetabular are all, except :**
A. Recurrent dislocations despite fixation with traction
B. Open acetabular fracture
C. Progressive sciatic nerve involvement
D. Morel-Lavallee lesion

536. Trigger finger is most likely to be associated with :
A. Diabetes B. Trauma
C. Gout D. Rheumatoid arthritis

Ans. 528. B 529. B 530. C 531. C 532. D 533. C
534. A 535. D 536. D

537. **Milkman's syndrome is :**
A. Radiological diagnosis
B. Acute osteomyelitis
C. Rheumatic arthritis
D. Pseudofracture with osteomalacia/rickets
E. Vitamin-A intoxication

538. **Rocker bottom feet are due to :**
A. Tuberculosis
B. Trauma
C. Actinomycosis
D. Maduramycosis
E. Over correction of equino deformity

539. **Compression of single vertebra with narrow joint space is characteristic of :**
A. Caries spine
B. Fracture spine
C. Prolapsed intervertebral disc
D. Secondaries spine

540. **Widening of intercondylar notch of femur is due to :**
A. Trauma
B. Hemophilia
C. Rheumatoid arthritis
D. Osteoarthritis
E. Ewing's tumor

541. **Allis sign is seen in :**
A. Osteochondritis
B. Marfan's syndrome
C. CDH
D. Osteoarthritis

542. **True about narrow lumbar canal syndrome are all, except :**
A. Claudication
B. Rotation of spine causes pain
C. Can be diagnosed only by myelography
D. May lead to spastic paraplegia
E. Due to congenital vertebral anomaly

543. **Foot drop occurs due to lesion in following, except :**
A. Common Peroneal nerve
B. L5 root
C. S1 root
D. Ant. tibial nerve

Ans. 537. D 538. E 539. A 540. B 541. C 542. E
543. D

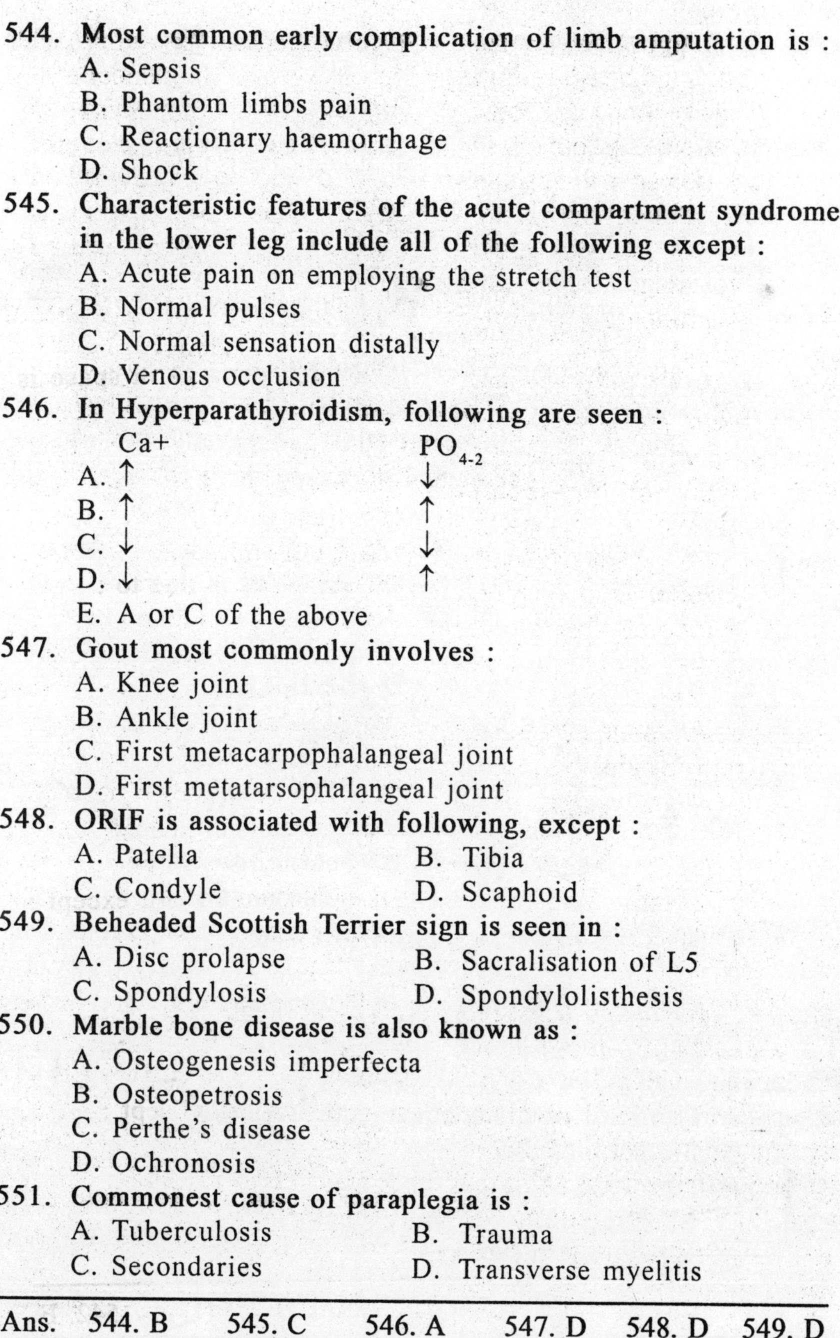

544. Most common early complication of limb amputation is :

A. Sepsis
B. Phantom limbs pain
C. Reactionary haemorrhage
D. Shock

545. Characteristic features of the acute compartment syndrome in the lower leg include all of the following except :

A. Acute pain on employing the stretch test
B. Normal pulses
C. Normal sensation distally
D. Venous occlusion

546. In Hyperparathyroidism, following are seen :

	Ca^{+}	$PO_{4^{-2}}$
A.	$\uparrow$	$\downarrow$
B.	$\uparrow$	$\uparrow$
C.	$\downarrow$	$\downarrow$
D.	$\downarrow$	$\uparrow$

E. A or C of the above

547. Gout most commonly involves :

A. Knee joint
B. Ankle joint
C. First metacarpophalangeal joint
D. First metatarsophalangeal joint

548. ORIF is associated with following, except :

A. Patella B. Tibia
C. Condyle D. Scaphoid

549. Beheaded Scottish Terrier sign is seen in :

A. Disc prolapse B. Sacralisation of L5
C. Spondylosis D. Spondylolisthesis

550. Marble bone disease is also known as :

A. Osteogenesis imperfecta
B. Osteopetrosis
C. Perthe's disease
D. Ochronosis

551. Commonest cause of paraplegia is :

A. Tuberculosis B. Trauma
C. Secondaries D. Transverse myelitis

Ans. 544. B 545. C 546. A 547. D 548. D 549. D
550. B 551. A

552. **Bleeding into joint cavities is not common in :**
A. Hemophilia B. ITP
C. Christmas disease D. None of the above

553. **Find out the wrong match :**
A. Hyperparathyroidism—subperiosteal erosion of phalanges.
B. Rickets—Triradiate pelvis.
C. Osteosarcoma—Multiple calcified secondaries in brain.
D. Osteoclastoma—Soap bubble appearance.

554. **A 9-years old child with arched palate has shoulders meeting in front of his chest. He has :**
A. Erb's palsy B. Cleidocranial dysostosis
C. Chondrosteodystrophy D. Cortical hyperostosis

555. **A patient with fractures of both femurs, and unconsciousness. The correct sequence of management is :**
I—Airway maintenance
II—I/V fluids
III—Blood
IV—Reduction by splint
A. I, II, III, IV B. IV, III, II, I
C. II, I, III, IV D. III, II, I, IV

556. **Osteitis is caused by :**
A. Toxoplasma B. Rubella
C. Syphilis D. CMV

557. **In Burton's disease, there is :**
A. Scurvy and Rickets B. Scurvy and Syphilis
C. Syphilis and Rickets D. Scurvy and Pellagra

558. **Most common cause of pressure sore in the foot in India is :**
A. Diabetes mellitus B. Syringomyelia
C. Leprosy D. Thorn prick

559. **Hand Schuller Christian disease, which is correct :**
A. Proliferation of reticuloendothelial cells
B. Foam cells seen
C. Punched-out lesions in X-ray
D. Diabetes insipidus and exophthalmous present
E. All are correct

Ans. 552. B 553. C 554. B 555. A 556. C 557. A
558. C 559. E

560. Kashin-Beck disease most often involves :
A. Wrist B. Ankle
C. Phalanges D. Knee

561. Aseptic necrosis arising out of circulatory causes are except :
A. Slipped femoral epiphysis
B. Perthes' disease
C. Caisson disease
D. Radiation necrosis
E. Cortisone

562. Aseptic necrosis as a result of metabolic factors is associated with all, except :
A. Mucopolysaccharidosis
B. Abnormal hemoglobin
C. Gaucher's disease
D. Alcoholism
E. Cortisone therapy

563. Plantar fasciitis :
A. Is caused by a bony spur on the plantar surface of the os calcis.
B. Is not associated with infection elsewhere in the body.
C. Is a type of Dupuytren's disease.
D. Can be relieved by supplying insoles.

564. The periosteal or cortical desmoid of Kimmelstiel is a lesion best described as :
A. Identical to the cortical defect of Hatcher
B. Identical to the cortical defect of Jaffe
C. A small non-ossifying fibroma
D. A dense fibrous lesion
E. A lesion with numerous giant cells

565. Which of the single most important step in the management of a case of gas gangrene:
A. Anti-gas-gangrene serum
B. Blood transfusion
C. Penicillin injections
D. Surgical debridement of the wound
E. Administration of hyperbaric oxygen

Ans. 560. C 561. E 562. A 563. D 564. D 565. D

566. In long-term therapy in vitamin-D resistant rickets, the best guide to safe treatment is :

A. Urinary phosphate excretion
B. Urinary calcium excretion
C. Serum alkaline phosphatase
D. Serum phosphate level
E. Serum calcium level

567. Spontaneous haemorrhage during anticoagulant therapy in a non-surgical patient may be expected if the prothrombin level drops below :

A. 0% B. 5%
C. 10% D. 20%
E. 25%

568. In a patient with hyperparathyroidism and a blood calcium of 14 mg as a result of parathyroid adenoma the blood calcium levels following surgical removal of adenoma :

A. Do not necessarily change.
B. Slowly return to normal over 2-3 weeks.
C. Return to normal usually within 24 hours.
D. Return to normal or slightly subnormal rapidly.
E. Drop almost once to subnormal levels and tetany results.

569. A patient with severe bone destruction as a result of hyperparathyroidism and a fracture through a cyst in the femur should, after recovery from parathyroid surgery, be treated :

A. Conservatively for the fracture.
B. By an open reduction to clear out the brown tumor and the defect filled-in with a bone graft.
C. By an open reduction, curettage, bone graft, and metallic internal fixation.
D. By simple curettage of the brown tumor and bone graft without internal fixation.
E. Supportive treatment only as these lesions do not heal.

Ans. 566. B 567. C 568. E 569. A

570. **Tendon rupture due to degenerative tendon weakness is thought to be the result of :**
   A. Excess wear and tear.
   B. Collagen disease and degeneration.
   C. Central artery of the tendon thrombosis.
   D. Changes that physiologically occur in all tendons with age.
   E. Increasing weight of the individual and sporadic exercise.

571. **Carcinoma cheek is best treated by :**
   A. Busulphan
   B. Cyclophosphamide
   C. Vinblastine
   D. Cisplatinum

572. **A patient, after developing facial injury complains of diplopia. He has :**
   A. Subdural haematoma
   B. Fracture superior orbital fissure
   C. Fracture zygomatic arch
   D. Hysteria

573. **Best way to diagnose the above patient is :**
   A. CT scan B. X-ray
   C. Hypnoanalysis D. Clinical examination

574. **Spastic paraplegia is not found in :**
   A. Cervical spondylosis
   B. Lead poisoning
   C. Syringomyelia
   D. Sup. saggital sinus thrombosis

575. **Osteomalacia is caused by :**
   A. Phenytoin B. Procainamide
   C. Steroids D. Hydralazines

576. **Which one should be given prime priority in the emergency treatment of the seriously injured sports-man :**
   A. Transport on a firm surface immediately
   B. Splintage of all fracture sites
   C. Maintenance of airway
   D. Application of tourniquet over the bleeding area

Ans. 570. C 571. D 572. C 573. B 574. B 575. A
576. C

577. **Emergency care of the unconscious players include all, except :**
   A. Never give fluids.
   B. After a minor head injury, trainer or captain should ask the player regarding current score or location of event to exclude confusion or disorientation.
   C. Player should be allowed to continue the game, if unconsciousness is only for a few seconds.
   D. Observe for lack of movement which may indicate paralysis.

578. **Adrenocorticosteroids in excess cause :**
   A. Osteoporosis
   B. Osteosclerosis
   C. Osteochondritis
   D. Endochondral ossification

579. **Fat embolism may follow :**
   A. Fracture of long bones
   B. Multiple injuries
   C. Fracture of the patella
   D. Surgical incision through the spine
   E. All of the above

580. **Which of the following is best related to fat embolism :**
   A. 20% of polytrauma
   B. 40% of bilateral fracture femur
   C. 90% of trauma
   D. Only 15%

581. **Treatment based on 'Gate theory' is :**
   A. Short wave diatherapy
   B. Ultrasound
   C. Electrical nerve stimulation
   D. Infra-red therapy

582. **Still's disease is :**
   A. Spastic diplegia
   B. Rheumatoid arthritis in childhood
   C. Rheumatoid arthritis in the elderly
   D. Post-traumatic bone formation in the lateral ligament of the knee

---

Ans. 577. C 578. A 579. A 580. B 581. C 582. B

583. **Osteophytes developing at the joint at Luscka characteristically compresses spinal nerves at :**
A. Intervertebral foramen
B. Anterior part of body
C. Posterior part of body
D. Paradural areas

584. **Pott's puffy tumour is :**
A. Puffness of face following Pott's fracture
B. Puffness of face due to allergic reaction
C. Pott's spine
D. Frontal osteomyelitis with overlying soft tissue swelling

585. **Swan neck deformity is a feature of :**
A. Syphilitic arthritis B. Gouty arthritis
C. Rheumatoid arthritis D. Osteoarthritis

586. **The calcification of meniscus on knee joint is seen in:**
A. Hyperparathyroidism B. Pseudogout
C. Renal osteodystrophy D. T.B.

587. **TNM staging of carcinoma maxilla with skin involvement and lymphadenopathy:**
A. T1N2M0 B. T2N1M0
C. T2N2M0 D. T2N1M1

588. **Blount's disease is :**
A. Tibia vara B. Genu valgum
C. Pes planus D. None of the above

589. **Which of the following is known as Charcot Marie tooth disease :**
A. Caries tooth
B. Pyorrhea
C. Peroneal muscular atrophy
D. Syphilitic arthritis

590. **In which of the following condition/s is patella at a level higher than normal :**
A. Osgood Schlatter's disease
B. Defective meniscus
C. Recurrent dislocation patella
D. Nail patella syndrome

Ans. 583. A 584. D 585. C 586. B 587. B 588. A
589. C 590. C

591. **Which of the following is not a feature of rickets :**
A. Triradiate pelvis
B. Frontal bossing
C. Enlargement of costochondral junctions
D. Clutton joints

592. **Following are sclerosing disorders of bone except :**
A. Osteopetrosis B. Melorheostosis
C. Osteitis fibrosa D. Caffey's

593. **Commonest cause of anterior compartment syndrome is :**
A. Fractures
B. Schirrhous carcinoma
C. Superficial injury to muscles
D. Operative trauma

594. **The bone most commonly affected by Gaucher's disease is the :**
A. Femur B. Skull
C. Humerus D. Cervical spine

595. **A recessive form of osteogenesis imperfecta may closely resemble:**
A. Alkaptonuria B. Cretinism
C. Hypophosphatasia D. Homocystinuria

596. **Painful arc syndrome may be due to :**
A. Supraspinatus tendinitis
B. Partial tear of supraspinatus tendon
C. Subacromial bursitis
D. Crack fracture in greater tuberosity of humerus
E. Any of the above

597. **Compound palmar ganglion is :**
A. Tuberculous affection of ulnar bursa
B. Pyogenic affection of ulnar bursa
C. Non-specific affection of ulnar bursa
D. Ulnar bursitis due to compound injury
E. None of the above

Ans. 591. D 592. C 593. A 594. A 595. C 596. E
597. A

598. **Osgood-Schlatter's disease is defined as :**
A. Traction injury of posterior epiphysis of Os calcis
B. Traction injury of lunate
C. Traction injury of tibial tubercle
D. Traction injury of capital femoral epiphysis

599. **The most common cause of backache in old age is :**
A. Spondylolisthesis
B. Spondylosis
C. Prolapsed intervertebral disc
D. Ankylosing spondylitis
E. T.B. spine

600. **Infraction is :**
A. A green stick fracture in children
B. A type of infarction of bone
C. A type of impacted fracture in adult
D. Another name for compound fracture

601. **Mseleni joint disease most often involves :**
A. Knee B. Wrist
C. Ankle D. Hip

602. **Disease common in Ticket clippers :**
A. Driller's wrist B. Spoon-player's wrist
C. Bass player's thumb D. Wicket keeper's hand

603. **Heberden's nodules are seen in :**
A. Osteoarthritis B. Rheumatiod arthritis
C. Rheumatic arthritis D. Psoriatic arthritis

604. **HAL B27 is associated with :**
A. Rheumatoid arthritis
B. Ankylosing spondylitis
C. Rheumatic arthritis
D. Gouty arthritis

605. **Calcification of menisci is seen in :**
A. Hyperparathyroidism
B. Pseudogout
C. Renal osteodystrophy
D. Acromegaly

Ans. 598. C 599. B 600. A 601. D 602. C 603. A
604. B 605. B

606. Corticosteroids in post-operative period can cause :
A. Decrease in infection
B. Increase in infection
C. Increase in healing
D. Decrease in healing

607. Multiple punched at lesions in skull are seen in :
A. Hypoparathyroidism B. Rickets
C. Carcinoma prostate D. Multiple myeloma

608. In rickets, not seen is :
A. Talipes equinovarus B. Genu valgum
C. Genu varus D. Bow legs

609. Behcet's syndrome is commonest in :
A. Knee B. Ankle
C. Hip D. Wrist

610. Subsequent to a fall, a young man is unable to lift injured upper limb. On inspection, the normal rounded contour of the shoulder is found to have been lost; the upper arm appears longer on the injured side and the acromion is prominent. The most likely diagnosis is :
A. Fracture neck of the humerus
B. Anterior dislocation of the shoulder
C. Posterior dislocation of the shoulder
D. Acromio-clavicular dislocation

611. A 30-years old mother of four children has been noticing a hard painless swelling in front of the neck during the past eight months, gradually increasing in size. On coming down the stairs, she suddenly felt excruciating pain in the left hip and fell down and could not get-up any more. The most likely diagnosis is :
A. Stress fracture neck of femur
B. Dislocation of hip
C. Pathological fracture of upper-end of femur
D. Slipped femoral epiphysis

612. SLE most commonly involves ——— spine.
A. Cervical B. Thoracic
C. Lumbar D. Sacral

Ans. 606. D 607. D 608. A 609. A 610. B 611. C
612. A

613. **A 'Febella' is :**
A. Bony loose body in the knee joint.
B. Calcification in the tibial collateral ligament after partial avulsion from the medial condyle of the femur.
C. Calcification of the lateral collateral ligament near its attachment to the lateral condyle of femur.
D. A sesamoid bone in the lateral head of the gastrocnemius.
E. A sesamoid bone in both sides of the head of the 1st metatarsal bone.

614. **Patchy calcification may be seen in :**
A. Chondrosarcoma
B. Osteosarcoma
C. Giant cell tumour
D. Ewing's tumour

615. **The cardinal feature of irritable hip is :**
A. Extreme pain
B. Limp
C. Pain referred to the knee
D. Muscles spasm
E. Limitation of all movements at their extreme

616. **Which of the following cysts is medially situated :**
A. Housemaid's knee
B. Clergyman' knee
C. Bursa anserina
D. Semimembranosusbursitis
E. Morrant Baker's cyst

617. **Pain at the neck of the 2nd metatarsal bone is often diagnostic of :**
A. Freiberg's disease
B. Stress fracture
C. Morton's metatarsalgia
D. Splitting osteochondritis

618. **Pain between the heads of the 3rd and 4th metatarsal radiating to the adjacent sides of the toes indicates :**
A. Stress fracture
B. Plantar fascitis
C. Morton's metatarsalgia
D. Sesamoid chondromalacia

Ans. 613. A 614. A 615. E 616. C 617. B 618. C

619. Which of the following has maximum malignant potential:
A. Perthes' disease
B. Paget's disease
C. Multiple chondromatosis
D. Aneurysmal bone cyst

620. Causes of painful limb are all, except :
A. Perthes disease
B. Congenital coxa vara
C. Slipped femoral epiphysis
D. TB hip

621. Commonest abnormality in rickets is :
A. Genu valgum B. Genu varum
C. Genu recurvatum D. Bow legs

622. Osteitis fibrosa cystica is seen in :
A. Hyperthyroidism
B. Hyperparathyroidism
C. Congenital bone disease
D. Hypoparathyroidism

623. Increased bone density is present in all except :
A. Osteopetrosis B. Metastasis from prostate
C. Fluorosis D. Hyperparathyroidism

624. Best result after repair of Flexor Tendon injuries of the hand occur if the injury is in :
A. Zone 1 B. Zone 2
C. Zone 3 D. Zone 4

625. Chondrolysis occurs commonly in :
A. Tuberculous arthritis
B. Septic arthritis of infancy
C. Syphilitic arthritis
D. Chondrosarcoma

626. Renal osteodystrophy does not include :
A. Osteomalacia B. Osteosclerosis
C. Osteoporosis D. Osteomyelitis

Ans. 619. B 620. B 621. A 622. B 623. D 624. B
625. C 626. D

627. Sub-periosteal erosions of middle phalanges at the radial aspect are characteristic of :

A. Hypothyroidism B. Hyperthyroidism
C. Hypoparathyroidism D. Hyperparathyroidism

628. After an operation of femur bone, chest X-ray shows widespread mottling throughout the lung field like a snowstorm. It is diagnostic of :

A. Fat embolism B. Shock lung
C. Bronchopneumonia D. Atelectasis

629. Vertebra plana is seen in :

A. TB
B. Eosinophilic granuloma
C. Trauma
D. Ankylosing spondylitis

630. Bone density is increased by :

A. Immobilisation
B. Postmenopausal
C. Parathyroid hormone
D. Estrogen in post-menopausal woman

631. Synovial membrane of knee joint, true is :

A. Continuous with prepatellar bursa
B. Continuous with intrapatellar bursa
C. Pierced by cruciate ligament posteriorly
D. Covers under surface of menisci

632. Intradistal pressure is least when a person is:

A. Standing B. Sitting
C. Lying supine D. Lying by side

633. How to differentiate gout with pseudogout :

A. Large joint involvement
B. Bifringent (particles) crystals
C. Serum uric acid normal
D. Associated with hyperparathyroidism

634. The integrity of palmar arch is tested by:

A. Allen's test B. Homan's test
C. Paget's test D. Schwartz's test

Ans. 627. D 628. A 629. B 630. D 631. C 632. C
633. B 634. D

635. Blood picture in a female - Ca.6mg%, uric acid- 14 mg% creatinine- 5 mg%, diagnosis is :
A. Rhabdomylosis
B. Acute uric acid nephropathy
C. Acute rheumatoid arthritis
D. Rickets

636. 8 years old child presented with fracture in the neck of humerus, one year back X-ray revealed cystic lesion, probable diagnosis is :
A. Unicameral bone cyst B. Osteomyelitis
C. Osteoclastoma D. Osteogenic sarcoma

637. Bankart's lesion is seen at :
A. Anterior surface of glenoid labrum
B. Posterior surface of glenoid labrum
C. Anterior part of head of humerus
D. Posterior part of head of humerus

638. In a 25 years old male with pain in upper part of left leg which is not relieved by rest but relieved by aspirin; probable diagnosis is :
A. Brodie's abscess B. Osteoid osteoma
C. Stress D. Rheumatoid arthritis

639. Carpal tunnel syndrome does not occur in :
A. Myopathy B. Pregnancy
C. Refsum's disease D. Colles' fracture

640. Main arterial supply of talus is by :
A. Dorsalis pedis artery B. Artery of sinus tarsi
C. Artery of tarsal canal D. Peroneal artery

641. In a tailor, hypoaesthesia and atrophy of thenar eminence is seen. The most likely nerve to be injured is :
A. Median nerve B. Radial nerve
C. Axillary nerve D. Ulnar nerve

642. Patient has pain on inner thigh with flexion, lat. rotation & adduction at hip. What is the site of lesion :
A. L1 B. L2
C. L3 D. L4
E. L5

Ans. 635. B 636. A 637. A 638. B 639. A 640. C 641. A 642. D

643. Pseudotumor is seen in :

A. Hemophilia B. AIDS
C. ITP D. Dermatomyositis

644. True about multiple epiphyseal dysgenesis is all, except :

A. Malignant transformation
B. Short bones
C. Pseudoarthrosis
D. Multiple swellings

645. Ganglion contains :

A. Mucoid material B. Blood
C. Water D. All of the above

646. Pseudoflexion deformity occurs due to :

A. Synovitis B. TB hip
C. Iliopsoasabscess D. Acetabular bursitis

647. Which activity will be difficult to perform for a patient with an anterior cruciate deficient knee joint :

A. Walk downhill B. Walk uphill
C. Sit cross-leg D. Getting-up from sitting

648. These ventral spinal rootlets are more prone to injury during decompressive operations because they are shorter and exist in a more horizontal direction :

A. C_5 B. C_6
C. C_7 D. T_1

649. A young motorist suffered injuries in a major road traffic accident. He was diagnosed to have fracture of left femur and left humerus. He was also having fractures of multiple ribs anteriorly on both the sides. On examination, the blood pressure was 80/60 mm Hg, and heart rate was 140/minute. The patient was agitated, restless, and tachypnic. Jugular veins were distended. Air entry was adequate in both the lung fields. Heart sounds were barely audible. Femoral pulses were weakly palpable but distally no pulsation could be felt. On priority basis, the immediate intervention would be :

A. Rapid blood transfusion
B. Urgent pericardial tap
C. Intercostal tube drainage on both the sides
D. Fixation of left femur and repair of femoral artery

Ans. 643. A 644. C 645. A 646. C 647. B 648. A 649. B

650. A 40-years-old man was repairing his wooden shed on Sunday morning. By afternoon, he felt that the hammer was becoming heavier and heavier. He felt pain in lateral side of elbow and also found that squeezing water out of sponge hurt his elbow. Which of the muscles are most likely involved :
A. Biceps brachii and supinator
B. Flexor digitorum superficialis
C. Extensor carpi radialis longus and brevis
D. Triceps branchii and anconeus

651. Following surgical removal of a firm nodular cancer swelling in the right breast and exploration of the right axilla. On examination the patient was found to have a winged right scapula. This occurred due to injury to the :
A. Subscapular muscle
B. Coracoid process of scapula
C. Long thoracic nerve
D. Circumflex scapular artery

652. A 49-years-old man suffering from carcinoma of prostate was X-rayed. He showed areas of sclerosis and collapse of T_{10} and T_{11} vertebrae in X-ray. The spread of this cancer to the above vertebrae was through :
A. Sacral canal
B. Lymphatic vessels
C. Internal vertebral plexus of veins
D. Superior rectal veins

653. All of the following are true about osteoporosis, except :
A. Milkmans fracture B. Bending of long bones
C. Hypercalcemia D. Vertebral compression fractures

654. Aseptic loosening in cemented total hip replacement, occurs as a result of hypersensitivity response to:
A. Titaneum debris
B. High density polythene debris
C. N, N-Dimethyltryptamine (DMT)
D. Free radicals

Ans. 650. C 651. C 652. C 653. C 654. B

655. Athletic pubalgia is due to :
A. Abdominal muscle strain
B. Quadriceps strain
C. Rectus femoris strain
D. Gluteus maximus strain

656. Recurrent dislocation is rare in :
A Ankle B. Hip
C. Shoulder D. Patella

657. Heberden's nodes are seen at the following joint :
A. Metacarpophalangeal
B. Distal Interphalangeal
C. Proximal Interphalangeal
D. Wrist

658. Least commonly seen in rheumatoid arthritis:
A. Peripheral neuropathy B. Raynaud's phenomenon
C. Pleural effusion D. Hepatomegaly

659. Following may occur in Marfan's syndrome, except :
A. Spontaneous pneumothorax
B. Striae over shoulders
C. Dolichostenomelia
D. Cataract

660. Precipitating factors in acute gouty arthritis include all of the following, except :
A. ACTH B. Roentgen therapy
C. Surgical procedure D. Alcohol

661. All are true of Ehler Danlos syndrome, except :
A. Long stature
B. Wide epicanthic fold
C. Elastic abnormal skin
D. Hypermobile joints

662. Which of the following statements about gout is false :
A. Acute attacks may be precipitated by weight reduction.
B. Olecranon bursitis is a recognised feature.
C. Premenopausal woman are rarely affected.
D. Thiazide diuretics will reduce the serum urate level.

Ans. 655. A 656. A 657. B 658. D 659. D 660. A
661. A 662. D

663. A 27-years-old woman presents with muscle weakness, ptosis, has been receiving gentamycin injections for the last seven days for a urinary infection. Thyroid function tests, serum creatine kinase, electromyogram and muscle biopsy are normal. Intravenous administration of edrophonium results in a dramatic improvement in the patient's muscle strength. Which of the following is the most likely diagnosis:

A. Duchenne muscular dystrophy
B. Myasthenia gravis
C. Toxic (drug-induced) myopathy
D. None of the above

664. The underlying pathology of the disease state of the patient is :

A. Inadequate acetylcholinesterase in the synaptic cleft.
B. Impaired synthesis/release of acetylcholine (Ach) in presynaptic vesicles.
C. Impaired release of Ach from presynaptic terminals.
D. Blockade of Ach receptors by autoantibodies.

665. Features more characteristic of the drug-induced form of systemic lupus than other cases of systemic lupus include :

A. Equal sex incidence
B. Kidney involvement
C. Fatal outcome
D. Low complement levels
E. Antibodies to native double strand DNA

666. It is likely that this patient's muscle weakness has been exacerbated by gentamycin through :

A. Inhibition of presynaptic release of Ach.
B. Potentiation of the action of acetylcholinesterase.
C. Increasing the turnover of Ach receptors.
D. Slowing the conduction of the action potential.

667. This adverse effect of aminoglycoside antibiotics can be antagonized by the intravenous administration of :

A. Calcium gluconate B. Copper sulphate
C. Magnesium phosphate D. None of the above

Ans. 663. B 664. D 665. A 666. A 667. A

668. A drug which prevents uric acid synthesis by inhibiting the enzyme xanthine oxidase is :

A. Probenecid B. Aspirin
C. Phenylbutazone D. Allopurinol
E. Colchicine

669. Sclerodermatous involvement of heart may lead to :

A. Cardiomyopathy B. Pericarditis
C. Heart block D. All of the above
E. None of the above

670. Which of the following drugs is known to cause muscle weakness that may be indistinguishable from that caused by the disease state of this patient :

A. Actinomycin B. Amoxycillin
C. Penicillamine D. Tetracycline

671. Sweaty feet syndrome is associated with :

A. G-6-P deficiency
B. Phenylalanine deficiency
C. Branched chain ketonuria
D. Isovaleric acidemia

672. SLE (Systemic Lupus Erythematosus) is mainly seen in :

A. Children B. Young males
C. Young females D. Elderly females

673. Neuropathic joints are not seen in :

A. Tabes dorsalis B. Leprosy
C. Diabetes mellitus D. Myopathy

674. Steinburg's sign in Marfan's syndrome is :

A. Recurrent dislocation of lens.
B. Long thumb i.e. when wrist is closed thumb protrudes out of wrist.
C. Typical echocardiographic finding of mitral regurgitation.
D. Laxity of joints.

675. Antibody specific for SLE is :

A. Anti RNA B. Anti SSDNA
C. Anti DSDNA D. Anti S m

Ans. 668. D 669. D 670. C 671. D 672. C 673. D 674. B 675. D

676. Enthesopathy is not seen in :
A. Rheumatoid arthritis B. Reiter's disease
C. Ankylosing spondylitis D. Psoriatic arthritis

677. All are features of Sjogren's syndrome, except :
A. Rarely associated with rheumatoid arthritis
B. Auto-antibodies may be present
C. Can be associated with myasthenia gravis
D. Manifestations are less serious than sicca syndrome

678. Following are complications of Rheumatoid arthritis, except :
A. Splenic infarcts B. Pericarditis
C. Endocarditis D. Polycythemia

679. Following are used in the treatment of acute gouty arthritis except :
A. Piroxicam B. Ibuprofen
C. Naproxen D. Aspirin

680. C-Reactive protein is not raised in :
A. Rheumatic fever
B. Active rheumatoid arthritis
C. Acute gout
D. Viral fever

681. Which of the following may be used in the treatment of acute gout :
A. Aspirin B. Pyrazinamide
C. Allopurinol D. Indomethacin

682. Joint involvement is characteristically symmetrical in :
A. Rheumatoid arthritis B. Psoriatic arthritis
C. Osteoarthritis D. A + B of the above
E. C + gout

683. Rheumatoid arthritis complicated by splenomegaly, febrile polyarthritis and leukopenia is frequently termed :
A. Sjogren's syndrome
B. Palindromic rheumatism
C. Stevens-Johnson's syndrome
D. Still's disease
E. Felty's syndrome

Ans. 676. A 677. A 678. D 679. D 680. D 681. D
682. A 683. E

684. **Characteristic feature(s) of Wegener's granulomatosis is (are), except :**
A. Terminal uraemia
B. Nodular pulmonary lesions
C. Intractable rhinits and sinusitis
D. Congestive heart failure

685. **A young woman with arthritis, Raynaud's phenomenon and dysphagia is most likely to have :**
A. Polyarteritis
B. Regional enteritis
C. Rheumatoid arthritis
D. Scleroderma
E. S.L.E.

686. **Polyarteritis nodosa frequently includes all of the following, except :**
A. Lymphadenopathy
B. Fever and leucocytosis
C. Asthmatic attacks
D. Glomerulonephritis
E. Peripheral neuropathy

687. **Females are more likely to have all, except :**
A. Ankylosing spondylitis
B. Heberden's nodes
C. Peripheral rheumatoid arthritis
D. Systemic lupus erythematosus

688. **Tay-Sach's disease is characterized by all of the following, except :**
A. Mucular degeneration
B. Ballooning of cerebral ganglion cells
C. Spasticity
D. Glycogen storage

689. **Raynaud's sphenomenon can occur in the cases of :**
A. Cervical rib
B. Cryoglobulinaemia
C. Collagen disease
D. Thromboangitis obliterans
E. All of the above

690. **The following are true of drug induced lupus, except :**
A. Renal and CNS involvement are common
B. Anti-DS DNA antibodies are rare
C. Hypocomplementemia is rare
D. Common in slow acetylators

Ans. 684. D 685. D 686. A 687. C 688. D 689. E 690. A

691. Wrong about gout is :
A. Ist metacarpophalangeal joint involved
B. Joint pain
C. Crystals (calcium pyrophosphate) in joint
D. Nephritis

692. The change seen in the muscular arteries in polyarteritis nodosa :
A. Plasma cell infiltration
B. Eosinophilic infiltration
C. Intimal proliferation
D. Multiple nodules

693. Migrating polyarthritis is seen in :
A. Rheumatic fever B. Osteoarthritis
C. Rheumatoid arthritis D. None of the above

694. Commonest involvement of spine in rheumatoid arthritis is at :
A. Cervical B. Thoracic
C. Lumbar D. Sacroiliac joint

695. Caplan's syndrome is a manifestation of :
A. SLE B. Rheumatoid arthritis
C. Both of the above D. None of the above

696. Rheumatoid factor may be found in all of the following except :
A. SLE B. Sarcoidosis
C. Rheumatoid arthritis D. Fanconi's syndrome

697. Rose Waaler test is positive in 100% cases of :
A. Rheumatoid arthritis
B. Systemic lupus erythematosus
C. Sjogren's syndrome
D. Sarcoidosis

698. Which of the following is likely in a person who has headache, fever, leucocytosis, elevated ESR, anaemia and polymyalgia rheumatica :
A. Lupus erythematosus B. Temporal arteritis
C. Scleroderma D. Migraine

Ans. 691. C 692. D 693. A 694. A 695. B 696. D
697. C 698. B

699. **Rheumatoid spondylitis is associated with :**
A. Aortic insufficiency
B. Aortic stenosis
C. Mitral insufficiency
D. Mitral stenosis

700. **A young female with Raynaud's phenomenon in hands with no other abnormality is suffering from :**
A. Carcinoid
B. Pseudoxanthoma elasticum
C. Progressive systemic sclerosis
D. Burger's disease

701. **Plucked chicken skin appearance is pathognomonic of :**
A. Pseudoxanthoma elasticum
B. Marfan's syndrome
C. Homocystinuria
D. Any of the above

702. **What percent of gouty individuals have nephrolithiasis :**
A. 10-20% B. 30-40%
C. 2-5% D. 50-60%

703. **Hartnup disease includes all, except :**
A. Psychosis
B. Cerebellar ataxia
C. Photosensitive dermatitis
D. Raised serotonin levels

704. **Cystinuria is commonly associated with :**
A. Homocystinuria
B. Hexagonal crystals in the urine
C. Severe mental retardation
D. All of the above

705. **Scleroderma may be associated with, except :**
A. Alveolar cell carcinoma
B. Peribronchial fibrosis, cor pulmonale
C. Recurrent bronchopneumonia due to aspiration
D. None of the above

Ans. 699. A 700. C 701. A 702. A 703. D 704. B 705. D

706. **A 20-years old female presents with fever, joint pains, skin rash, anaemia, haematurea and high ESR (120 mm/hr). The most likely diagnosis is :**
A. Acute rheumatic fever
B. Acute glomerulonephritis
C. Systemic lupus erythematosus
D. Polyarteritis nodosa

707. **Which is the most common site of sub-cutaneous nodules in rheumatoid arthritis :**
A. Elbow B. Wrist
C. Achilles tendon D. Occiput

708. **Which muscle is not involved in Duchenne's muscular dystrophy :**
A. Infraspinatus B. Brachioradialis
C. Vastus medialis D. Gastronemius

709. **Which is not seen in myasthenia gravis :**
A. Proximal involvement B. Symptoms on exertion
C. Remissions occur D. Absent DTR

710. **False about dermatomyositis is :**
A. Myoglobinuria
B. Patchy infiltration on biopsy
C. Ocular involvement
D. EMG diagnostic

711. **Polymyositis does not involve :**
A. Ocular muscles B. Pharyngeal muscles
C. Neck muscles D. Proximal muscles

712. **Consider the following statements about rheumatoid factor :**
1. It is uniformly present in patients with rheumatoid vasculitis.
2. It is a good screening test for the diagnosis of rheumatoid arthritis.
3. High titres predict a progressive course of the disease in rheumatoid arthritis with severe extra-articular manifestations.
4. The presence of rheumatoid factor is not specific for rheumatoid arthritis.

Of these statements
A. 1, 2 and 4 are correct B. 2 and 3 are correct
C. 3 and 4 are correct D. 1, 3 and 4 are correct

Ans. 706. C 707. A 708. A 709. D 710. C 711. A 712. D

713. **In Niemann-Pick disease, reticuloendothelial cells of liver are infiltrated with :**
A. Kerasin
B. Sphingomyelin
C. Cholesterol
D. Glycogen
E. Copper

714. **Osteogenesis imperfecta is characterized by all of the following, except :**
A. Blue sclerae
B. Multiple
C. Cataracts
D. Progressive deafness
E. Loose-jointedness

715. **Gout first involves :**
A. Knee joint
B. Ankles
C. Ist metatarsophalangeal joint
D. Ist metacarpophalangeal joint

716. **Still's disease is characterised by all, except :**
A. Cervical spondylitis
B. Lymphadenopathy
C. Pleuritis
D. Test for rheumatoid factor usually positive

717. **X-ray findings in degenerative joint disease, osteoarthritis include all, except :**
A. Bony sclerosis
B. Marginal lipping
C. Osteoporosis
D. Narrowing of joint space

718. **Oesophageal involvement in scleroderma :**
A. Atrophy of muscularis
B. Decreased collagen content
C. Involves upper-one-third
D. Does not affect mucosa

719. **Malignancy is classically associated with :**
A. Polyarteritis
B. Dermatomyositis
C. Scleroderma
D. Systemic lupus erythematosus

720. **Sjogren's syndrome involves all, except :**
A. Malignant lymphoma
B. Rheumatoid arthritis
C. Xerophthalmia
D. Xerostomia

Ans. 713. B 714. C 715. C 716. D 717. C 718. C
719. B 720. A

721. **Lesion most typical of rheumatoid arthritis is :**
A. Erythema multiforme
B. Erythema nodosum
C. Subcutaneous nodule
D. Erythema induratum

722. **Pseudogout can be distinguished from gout by means of :**
A. Acute onset
B. Positive birefringent crystals
C. Association with diabetes mellitus
D. Involvement of large joints

723. **One of the following is not part of picture of sclero-derma :**
A. Arthritis
B. Dysphagia
C. Diffuse calcinosis
D. Pathological fractures

724. **Characteristics of phenylketonuria include all of the following, except :**
A. Light colour of hair and skin
B. Excretion of phenyl pyruvic acid in urine
C. Hypocalcaemia
D. Mental retardation
E. Seizures

725. **Enzyme studies in glycogen storage disease may be easily performed on :**
A. Blood leukocytes
B. Blood platelets
C. Buccal mucosal cells
D. Testicular cells

726. **Homocystinuria does not affect the :**
A. Bones
B. Eyes
C. Bone marrow
D. CNS

727. **Excretion of homogentisic acid in urine is seen in :**
A. Cystic fibrosis
B. Galactosemia
C. Phenylketonuria
D. Alkaptonuria

728. **Rheumatoid arthritis is most often associated with the antigens :**
A. DR 4 and DR1
B. DR 3 and DR 5
C. B 27 and DR 5
D. DW 3 and DR 5

Ans. 721. C 722. B 723. D 724. C 725. D 726. C
727. D 728. A

729. **A 30-years old female with rheumatoid arthritis of five years duration complains of pain in the first three fingers of her right hand over the past six weeks. The pain seems especially severe at night often awakening her from sleep. The most likely cause of this patient's complaint is :**
A. Atlanto-axial sublaxation of cervical spine
B. Sensory peripheral neuropathy
C. Carpal Tunnel syndrome
D. Rheumatoid vasculitis

730. **Ankylosing spondylitis is usually associated with :**
A. Peripheral arthritis usually involving large joints (knees, ankles, hips etc).
B. Heal pain is common.
C. Characteristic involvement of sacroiliac joint.
D. Deformity of peripheral joints is uncommon.
E. All of the above.

731. **Which is associated with hypertension most prominently :**
A. Hurler's syndrome
B. Marfan's syndrome
C. Pseudoxanthoma elastica
D. Ehler's Danlos syndrome

732. **Features of Morquio's disease may include all of the following, except :**
A. Mental retardation.
B. Vertebrae are flattened.
C. Exaggerated thoracic kyphosis.
D. Abnormal amounts of kerato sulphate may be excreted in the urine.
E. Osseous development may appear normal until the infant begins to walk.

733. **Pseudogout has been associated with or encountered in :**
A. Ochronosis
B. Haemochromatosis
C. Diabetes mellitus
D. Hyperparathyroidism
E. All of the above

Ans. 729. C 730. E 731. C 732. A 733. E

734. **A finding not seen in dermatomyositis is :**
A. Creatinuria
B. Myoglobinuria
C. Raised SGOT
D. Depressed alpha-2-globulin

735. **Basic defect in genetic mucopolysaccharidosis is :**
A. Abnormal lysosomal enzymes
B. Excess iron in tissues
C. Abnormal elastic tissues
D. Insulin deficiency

736. **Systemic lupus erythematosus occurs most commonly in :**
A. Children
B. Elderly men
C. Elderly women
D. Women of child bearing age

737. **The most common toxic reactions of gold therapy in the treatment of rheumatoid arthritis include :**
A. Agranulocytosis
B. Dermatitis and stomatitis
C. Nausea and vomiting
D. Alopecia
E. Thrombophlebitis

738. **Patient with normal eyes and skin has defect of phenylalanine metabolism. There is increased excretion of hydroxyphenyl pyruvate in urine. Condition is :**
A. Alkaptonuria
B. Phenylketonuria
C. Tyrosinosis
D. Albinism

739. **Sicca syndrome is associated with :**
A. Rheumatoid arthritis
B. Laennec's cirrhosis
C. Scleroderma
D. SLE

740. **Rheumatoid factor may be seen in all, except :**
A. Typhoid
B. Syphilis
C. Pulmonary tuberculosis
D. Infectious mononucleosis

741. **True about drug induced systemic lupus erythematosis is :**
A. It is most often caused by Procainamide.
B. Rarely disappears on discontinuation of drug.
C. Has better prognosis as compared to idiopathic type.
D. Antinuclear antibodies are absent.

Ans. **734. D** **735. A** **736. D** **737. B** **738. A** **739. A**
740. A **741. C**

742. **Cardiac lesion commonly associated with rheumatoid arthritis is :**
A. Aortic stenosis
B. Mitral stenosis
C. Mitral incompetence (regurgitation)
D. Aortic regurgitation

743. **A patient with rheumatoid arthritis is not responding to routine treatment. Which one of the following is not to be indicated in further treatment :**
A. Methotrexate B. Salazopyrin
C. Endoxan D. Paracetamol

744. **Periungual telangiectasia are not seen in :**
A. Systemic lupus erythematosus
B. Dermatomyositis
C. Leprosy
D. Scleroderma

745. **Farr test is used to detect anti DNA antibodies in :**
A. Multiple myeloma B. Dermatomyositis
C. Purpura D. SLE

746. **Bluish color of sclera in osteogenesis imperfecta is due to :**
A. Thinness of collagen B. Deposition of pigment
C. Deposition of mucin D. All of the above

747. **Uricosuric drug is :**
A. Indometacin B. Probenecid
C. Colchicine D. Allopurinol

748. **Ankylosing spondylitis is associated with :**
A. HLA B27 B. HLA DR 4
C. HLA B8 D. HLA A3

749. **Raynaud's phenomenon, generalized calcinosis and dysphagia is seen in :**
A. Scleroderma B. SLE
C. Rheumatoid arthritis D. Cysticercosis

750. **Following is an omnious sign in osteogenesis imperfecta :**
A. Accordian femora
B. Beaded ribs
C. "Popcorn like" deposits at the end of long bones
D. Multiple fractures

Ans. 742. C 743. B 744. C 745 D 746. A 747. B
748. A 749. A 750. C

751. The commonest site for amyloid deposit is :
A. Lungs B. Large bowel
C. Heart D. Tongue

752. All are true about hypokalemic periodic paralysis, except :
A. Autosomal dominant
B. Decreased serum 'K' level
C. Muscle biopsy showing presence of vacuoles
D. Sodium channel defect

753. Maple syrup urine disease has the following amino acids in urine, except :
A. Leucine B. Isoleucine
C. Lysin D. Valine

754. Remmission inducing drugs or disease modifying drugs for rheumatoid arthritis include:
A. Aspirin B. Ibuprofen
C. Gold Thiol D. Naproxen

755. "Skipped generations" due to variable expressivity is common in :
A. Ehlers-Danlos syndrome
B. Osteogenesis imperfecta
C. Marfan's syndrome
D. Wilson's disease

756. Seronegative arthritis include :
A. Ankylosing spondylitis B. Reiter's arthritis
C. Psoriatic arthritis D. Enteropathic arthritis
E. All of the above

757. The best drug for treating SLE is :
A. Aspirin B. Indomethacin
C. Phenylbutazone D. Depinin
E. Steroids

758. Before starting a patient of SLE on long term glucocorticoid therapy, pre-treatment evaluation should include all except :
A. Chest X-ray and Tuberculin test
B. ACTH infusion test
C. Stool test for occult blood
D. Thoracic and lumbar spine films

Ans. 751. B 752. D 753. C 754. C 755. C 756. E
757. E 758. B

759. **Which one of the following is associated with CREST (Calcinosis, Raynaud's phenomenon, Oesophageal hypomotility, Sclerodactyly and Telangiectasia) syndrome :**
A. Systemic lupus erythematosis
B. Dermatomyositis
C. Polyarteritis nodosa
D. Progressive systemic sclerosis

760. **Schober's sign is :**
A. Flexion of lumbar spine
B. Chest expansion
C. Pain with motion of hip
D. Neck pain & stiffness

761. **All are seen in SLE, except :**
A. Pterygium B. Alopecia
C. Anaemia D. Arthritis

762. **In rheumatoid arthritis, which of the following is not seen :**
A. Coronary arteritis B. Pericarditis
C. Aortic dilatation D. Endocarditis

763. **A 35 years old business man presents suddenly with severe pain, swelling and redness in left big toe in early morning. Most likely diagnosis is :**
A. Rheumatoid arthritis B. Gouty arthritis
C. Pseudogout D. Septic arthritis

764. **Which of the following is most strongly associated with anti-mitochondrial antibody and anti-cytoplasmic antibody :**
A. Rheumatoid arthritis
B. SLE
C. Chronic active hepatitis
D. Primary biliary cirrhosis

765. **RA factor is used mainly in :**
A. Screening are patients for rheumatoid artheritis
B. Predicting multisystem disease
C. Predicting severity of disease
D. Monitoring treatment

Ans. 759. D 760. A 761. A 762. D 763. B 764. C
765. C

766. Corticosteroids are indicated in PSS with :

A. Myositis B. Esophageal dysmotitis
C. Pulmonary fibrosis D. Renal involvement

767. Which of the following collagen vascular diseases is not commonly associated with pulmonary fibrosis :

A. SLE B. PSS
C. Dermatomyositis D. Rheumatoid arthritis

768. Which of the following is associated with double stranded DNA antibody:

A. Juvenile RA B. SLE
C. RA D. PSS

769. Which about Gout is not true :

A. Acute attack may be seen in absence of causes.
B. Seen best by polarising light microscope.
C. Patient may be asymptomatic (with increased uric acid) for year.
D. Development of arthritis co-relates well with level of uric acid.

770. Which of the following is associated with an anti-body against an isolated antigen :

A. SLE B. MCTD
C. Sarcoidosis D. PSS

771. In Marfan's syndrome, aortic aneurysm occurs in :

A. Ascending aorta B. Descending thoracic aorta
C. Abdominal aorta D. Arch of aorta

772. Match List-I with List-II and select the correct answer using the codes given below the lists :

List-I (Disease)	List-II (Serological markers)
I. Mixed connective tissue disease	(i) ds-DNA antibodies
II. Renal lupus	(ii) HLA-B27
III. Reiter's syndrome	(iii) Anti-RNP antibodies
IV. Polyarteritis nodosa	(iv) Hbs Ag

Ans. 766. A 767. ALL 768. B 769. D 770. B 771. A
772. D

Codes :

A. I (iii)	II (i)	III (iv)	IV (ii)
B. I (i)	II (iii)	III (iv)	IV (ii)
C. I (i)	II (iii)	III (ii)	IV (iv)
D. I (iii)	II (i)	III (ii)	IV (iv)

773. **Mononeuritis multiplex is recognised complication of all of the following, except :**
A. Rheumatoid arthritis B. Polyarteritis nodosa
C. Diabetes mellitus D. Psoriatic arthropathy

774. **Type-V of Ehlers-Danlos syndrome is similar to type--------- but characterized by X-linked inheritance.**
A. I B. II
C. IV D. VII
E. VIII

775. **When will you suspect polyarteritis nodosa :**
A. Hypertension with mononeuritis
B. Hypertension with anemia
C. GN with hypergammaglobulinemia
D. All of the above

776. **Incidence of Raynaud's phenomenon is lowest with :**
A. SLE B. Rheumatoid arthritis
C. Sjogren's syndrome D. Myositis

777. **The following enzyme is not elevated in polymyositis :**
A. Creatine kinase B. Aldolase
C. Lactate dehydrogenase D. Amylase

778. **The earliest muscle to be involved in dermato-myositis is :**
A. Deltoid B. Gluteal
C. Lumbricals D. Quadriceps

779. **Disease modifying antirheumatic drugs are all, except:**
A. Nimesulide B. Azathioprine
C. Chloroquine D. Sulphasalazine

780. **Rhabdomyolysis occurs in :**
A. Volume depletion B. Cocaine overdosage
C. Hyperphosphatemia D. None of the above

Ans. 773. D 774. B 775. D 776. B 777. D 778. A
779. A 780. A

781. **True about polymyositis is :**
A. Ocular muscle involvement
B. Pharyngeal involvement
C. Muscle atrophy
D. Brisk reflexes common

782. **Neuro-cutaneous syndromes associated with CNS tumours are all, except :**
A. Tuberous sclerosis
B. von Hippel-Lindau
C. Sturge-Weber
D. Neurofibromatosis

783. **Extraglandular primary Sjogrens, syndrome is caused by following, except :**
A. SO_2
B. Lead
C. Asbestos
D. Silica

784. **True about Sarcoidosis is :**
A. Kvein test is not used for diagnosis
B. Pleural effusion seen
C. Associated with ANA
D. Common in males

785. **A 20-years old woman presents with history of recurrent pain in abdomen and appendicostomy two years back. She develops acute altered sensorium following a generalized tonic-clonic convulsions. On examination, the patient is drowsy and confused. She also has quadriparesis and all deep tendon reflexes are absent. Blood parameters, CSF examination and cranial CT are normal. The most likely diagnosis is :**
A. Hypertensive encephalopathy
B. Acute intermittent porphyria
C. Acute infective polyneuritis
D. Systemic lupus erythematosus

786. **True about Gaucher's disease are all, except :**
A. β-Glucocerebrosidease deficiency
B. No neurologic symptoms in adult form
C. Angiokeratomas
D. Autosomal dominant inheritance

Ans. 781. B 782. A 783. NONE 784. A 785. B
786. D

787. Homocystinuria resembles :
A. Mucopolysaccharidosis-II
B. Mucopolysaccharidosis-IV
C. Marfan's syndrome
D. Ehlers-Danlos syndrome

788. Ramesh 60 years, presents with generalized bone pain. On examination there is elevated ESR of 100 mm, serum globulin 7, lytic lesions in the skull, serum creatinine of 3.5 mg/dL and serum calcium of 11 mg/dL. What is the most likely diagnosis:
A. Waldenstrom's macroglobulinemia
B. Multiple myeloma
C. Hyperparathyroidism
D. Osteomalacia

789. Gout induced nephropathy earliest manifest as :
A. HT B. Isothenuria
C. ARF D. Pyelonephritis

790. Lyme disease stage-III, feature is :
A. Arthritis B. Myocarditis
C. CNS involvement D. Rash

791. Serum CK levels are low in myopathy associated with :
A. Hyperthyroidism B. Hypothyroidism
C. Hyperparathyroidism D. Hypoparathyroidism

792. In myasthenia gravis, correct statement regarding thymectomy is :
A. Done in all cases between puberty and 55 years of age.
B. Done in cases with ocular involvement only.
C. Not required if controlled by anticholinesterases.
D. Most cases are associated with thymoma.

793. In SLE all are seen, except :
A. Abortions B. Stillbirths
C. Conduction blocks D. Sterility

794. In rheumatoid arthritis all are seen, except :
A. High fever
B. Anorexia & weight loss
C. Affects age gap 40-60
D. Joint pain & swelling seen

Ans. 787. C 788. B 789. A 790. A 791. A 792. A
793. C 794. A

795. **All are causes of seronegative polyarthritis with ocular manifestations, except :**
   A. Psoriatic arthritis
   B. Behcet's arthritis
   C. Rheumatoid arthritis
   D. Inflammatory bowel disease associated arthritis

796. **Synovial fluid examination in rheumatoid arthritis will show :**
   A. Polymorphonuclear leucocytosis
   B. Decreased sugar content
   C. Cloudy in appearance
   D. Decreased complement levels

797. **Proximal muscle weakness is seen in all, except :**
   A. Duchenne's muscular dystrophy
   B. Myotonic dystrophy
   C. Spinal muscular dystrophy
   D. Myasthenia gravis

798. **In alkaptonuria, pigmentation is not seen in :**
   A. Ears B. Eyes
   C. Nose D. Articular cartilage

799. **Rheumatoid factor in rheumatoid arthritis is important because :**
   A. RA factor is associated with bad prognosis.
   B. Absent RA factor rules out the diagnosis of rheumatoid arthritis.
   C. It is very common in childhood rheumatoid arthritis.
   D. It correlates with disease activity.

800. **A 10 years old child presents with anemia and recurrent fractures. The X-ray shows diffuse hyperdensity of bone. The diagnosis is most likely to be :**
   A. Osteogenesis imperfecta
   B. Osteopetrosis
   C. Osteochondroma
   D. Hyperparathyroidism

Ans. 795. C 796. A 797. D 798. B 799. A 800. B

801. Lung involvement is seen in :
A. Polyarteritis nodosa
B. Henoch-Schonlein purpura
C. Cryoglobulinemic vasculitis
D. Wegener's granulomatosis

802. A patient presents with respiratory symptoms i.e. cought hemoptysis and glomerulonephritis. His c-ANCA levels in serum were found to be raised. The most likely diagnosis is :
A. Good pasture's syndrome
B. Classic polyarteritis nodosa
C. Wegener's granulomatosis
D. Kawasaki syndrome

803. A 20 years old woman presents with bilateral conductive deafness, palpable purpura on the legs and hemoptysis. Radiograph of the chest shows a thin-walled cavity in left lower zone. Investigations reveal total leukocyte count 12000/mm^3, red cell casts in the urine and 12000/mm^3 serum creatinine 3 mg/dL. What is the most probable diagnosis :
A. Henoch-Schonlein purpura
B. Polyarteritis nodosa
C. Wegener's granulomatosis
D. Disseminated tuberculosis

804. An 18 years old boy presents with digital gangrene in third and fourth fingers for last 2 weeks. On examination the blood pressure is 170/110 mm Hg and all peripheral pulses were palpable. Blood and urine examinations were unremarkable. Antinuclear antibodies, antibody to double stranded DNA and antineutrophil cytoplasmic antibody were negative. The most likely diagnosis is :
A. Wegener's granulomatosis
B. Polyarteritis nodosa
C. Takayasu's arteritis
D. Systemic lupus erythematosus (SLE)

805. Which one of the following is least likely to occur in late extra articular sero-positive rheumatoid arthritis :
A. Neutropenia B. Dry eye
C. Leg ulcers D. Hepatitis

Ans. 801. D 802. C 803. C 804. B 805. D

806. Which one of the following is not an X-linked recessive muscular dystrophy :
A. Duchenne muscular dystrophy
B. Becker's muscular dystrophy
C. Limb Girdle muscular dystrophy
D. Emergy-Dreifuss muscular dystrophy

807. Commonest complication of SLE is :
A. Haematological B. Renal
C. Liver (Hepatic) D. CNS

808. Which one of the following is correct regarding Eaton-Lambert syndrome :
A. It commonly affects the ocular muscles.
B. Neostigmine is the drug of choice for this syndrome.
C. Repeated electrical stimulation enhances muscle power in it
D. It is commonly associated with adenocarcinoma of lung.

809. A patient presents with melaena, normal renal function, hypertension and mononeuritis multiplex. The most probable diagnosis is :
A. Classical polyarteritis nodosa
B. Microscopic polyangitis
C. Henoch Schonlein purpura
D. Buerger's disease

810. A 30 years old male patient presents with complaints of weakness in right upper and both lower limbs for last 4 months. He developed digital infarcts involving 2nd and 3rd fingers on right side and 5th finger on left side. On examination, BP was 160/140 mm Hg, all peripheral pulses were palpable and there was asymmetrical neuropathy. Investigations showed a Hb 12 gm, TLC - 12000 Cu mm, Platelets 4,30,000, ESR-49 mm. Urine examination showed proteinuria and RBC - 10-15 hpf with no casts. Which of the following is the most likely diagnosis :
A. Polyarteritis nodosa
B. Systemic lumpus erythematosus
C. Wegener's granulomatosis
D. Mixed cryoglobulemia

Ans. 806. C 807. A 808. C 809. A 810. A

811. **Heberden's arthropathy affects :**
A. Lumber spine
B. Symmetrically large joints
C. Sarcoiliac joints
D. Distal interphalangeal joints

812. **The most sensitive test for the diagnosis of myasthenia gravis is :**
A. Elevated serum ACh-receptor binding antibodies
B. Repetitive nerve stimulation test
C. Positive edrophonium test
D. Measurement of jitter by single fibre electromyography

813. **False-positive rheumatoid factor can be associated with all, except :**
A. Inflammatory bowel disease
B. HbsAG
C. VDRL
D. Coobs test

814. **A young man with gout synovial fluid removed. It would shows :**
A. MSU crystals
B. CPPD crystals
C. PMN cells
D. Mono nuclear cells

815. **The chances of having an unaffected baby, when both parents have achondroplasia, are:**
A. 0%
B. 25%
C. 50%
D. 100%

816. **"Joint mice" are seen in :**
A. Osteogenic sarcoma
B. Enchondroma
C. Rheumatoid arthritis
D. Osteoarthritis

817. **Sometimes bone-formation is seen to follow an injury to a soft tissue, it could be due to :**
A. Calcification
B. Metaplasia
C. Dysplasia
D. Abnormal hypertrophy

818. **Synovial fluid has the following characteristics, except :**
A. Viscid and clear
B. Less than 2,000 cells/mm^3
C. Mucin
D. Fibrinogen

Ans. 811. D 812. D 813. A 814. A 815. B 816. D
817. B 818. D

819. In Juvenile Rheumatoid arthritis, all of the following are seen except:

A. Increased ESR
B. Polymorphonuclear leucocytosis
C. Positive latex fixation
D. Positive Bentonite floculation
E. Raised ASO litre

820. Rheumatic nodules are :

A. Painful
B. Attached to skin
C. Commoner in adults than children
D. Rarely occur unless active carditis is there

821. Common sites for osseous type of hydatid cysts are all, except:

A. Femur B. Skull
C. Vertebrae D. Ribs

822. Rheumatoid factor may be positive in all of the following, except :

A. Primary syphilis
B. TB
C. Enteric fever
D. Infectious mononucleosis

823. "————licks the joint, but bites the heart" :

A. Rheumatism
B. Synovitis
C. Fracture of bony end
D. Haemorrhage into the joint

824. Calcification front in a bone biopsy can be visualised by using stain :

A. Solochrome-cyanin-R
B. Alizarin-Red-S
C. Von Kossa
D. Masson's trichrome

825. Woven bone is found in all of the following, except :

A. Fracture callus B. Fetal bones
C. Hyperparathyroidism D. Vitamin-D intoxication

Ans. 819. E 820. D 821. B 822. C 823. A 824. A 825. D

826. **All of the following stimulate proliferation of osteoclasts, except :**
A. Prostagiandin B. Parathromone
C. Vitamin-C D. None of the above

827. **Which Bone tumour is hormone dependent :**
A. Osteogenic sarcoma B. Ewings sarcoma
C. Osteoclastoma D. Fibrous dysplasia

828. **Myositis ossificans may be histologically confused with :**
A. Osteoblastoma B. Osteosarcoma
C. Osteoma D. Osteoid osteoma

829. **Common manifestation of both rheumatoid and osteoarthritis is :**
A. Increased ESR
B. Involvement of proximal interphalangeal joint
C. Anaemia
D. General muscular atrophy

Match the following (Ques 939-943)
A. Rheumatoid arthritis B. Osteoarthritis
C. Gouty arthritis D. Pyogenic arthritis
E. Osteoporosis

830. **Erosion of articular cartilage**
831. **Nodules (Heberden's nodes) at base of terminal phalanges**
832. **Thinning of cortical and trabecular bone**
833. **Frequent with estrogen deficiency**
834. **Foreign body giant cell reaction**

835. **Presence of osteoid without mineralization is seen in :**
A. Rickets B. Scurvy
C. Osteopetrosis D. Paget's disease

836. **Garr's osteomyelitis commonly involves:**
A. Jaw B. Femur
C. Ribs D. Small muscles of hand

837. **Autoimmune arthritis is seen in :**
A. Rheumatoid arthritis B. Osteoarthritis
C. Psoriatic arthritis D. Suppurative arthritis

Ans. 826. C 827. D 828. B 829. B 830. B 831. B
832. E 833. E 834. C 835. A 836. A 837. A

838. **All are giant cell lesions of bone, except :**
A. Aneurysmal bone cyst
B. Chondroblastoma
C. Brown tumor
D. Chondroma

839. **The dead bone seen in chronic osteomyelitis is :**
A. Sequestrum B. Involucrum
C. Sinus debris D. Cloaca

840. **All of the following are markers of bone resorption, except :**
A. Tartarate resistant acid phosphatase
B. Osteocalcin
C. Cross-linked N-telopeptide
D. Urine total free deoxypyridinoline

841. **Specific marker for synovial sarcoma is :**
A. T (X, 18) B. T (9, 22)
C. T (17-9) D. T (11, 14)

842. **Stain of mineralization of newly formed osteoid :**
A. von Kossa stain B. Alizarin red
C. Labeled tetracycline D. Fluorescence

843. **Subperiosteal erosions of middle phalanges on the radial aspect is characteristic of :**
A. Hypoparathyroidism B. Hyperparathyroidism
C. Hyperthyroidism D. Hypothyroidism

844. **In bone infarcts, all are true except :**
A. In dysbaric osteonecrosis are commonly in juxtaarticular
B. Occurs in Gaucher's disease
C. Occurs in thalassaemia major
D. Are often diaphyseal in sickle cell disease
E. Are seen in acute pancreatitis

845. **Eccentric subarticular radiolucent lesion in ends of long bones is suggestive of :**
A. Osteoclastoma B. Osteogenic sarcoma
C. Aneurysmal bone cyst D. Osteoid osteoma

Ans. 838. D 839. A 840. B 841. A 842. C 843. B
844. A 845. C

846. **Dead bone on X-ray looks :**
A. Highly radio-opaque
B. Radio-opaque
C. Radiolucent
D. Not seen

847. **All are features of achondroplasia, except :**
A. Short and wide bones
B. Lumbar canal stenosis
C. Square shaped iliac bones
D. Flattening of vertebral body

848. **Which of the following is not a feature of Osteoge-nesis imperfecta :**
A. Thin and fragile bones B. Blue sclera
C. Otosclerosis D. Metaphyseal fracture

849. **The number of carpal bones seen in a radiograph of an infant is :**
A. 0 B. 2
C. 3 D. 5
E. 6

850. **Bone within bone vertebra may be seen in following, except :**
A. Rickets B. Scurvy
C. Hypothyroidism D. Hypoparathyroidism
E. Sickle cell anemia

851. **Age determination of a 18-years old on X-ray can be done from:**
A. Wrist B. Ankle
C. Knee D. Shoulder

852. **Widespread patchy sclerosis of the skeleton can be seen in, except :**
A. Mast cell reticulosis B. Carcinoma of the breast
C. Neuroblastoma D. Fluorosis
E. Myeloid metaplasia

853. **Radiostrontium bone scans have been found positive in :**
A. Fracture B. Bone tumours
C. Paget's disease D. All are true

Ans. 846. A 847. D 848. D 849. A 850. E 851. A
852. C 853. D

854. **Finding the non-union of the mandibular halves and of the zygomatic arches suggests :**
A. Arachnoidactyly
B. Cleidocranial dysostosis
C. Osteogenesis imperfecta
D. Morquio's disease

855. **X-ray examination in 'pulled elbow' usually shows :**
A. Dislocation
B. Subluxation
C. Radial head fracture
D. No osseous abnormality

856. **Onion peel appearance is seen in :**
A. Osteoclastoma B. Chondrosarcoma
C. Osteosarcoma D. Ewing's sarcoma

857. **Osteoporosis is diagnosed by all, except :**
A. Ultrasonography B. CT scan
C. Radiogammametry D. Plain X-ray

858. **Lytic lesion in upper end of tibia is expansile and has soap-buble appearance :**
A. Osteoclastoma B. Osteogenic sarcoma
C. Ewing's sarcoma D. Osteoblastoma

859. **Bifid manubrium may be seen in :**
A. Marfan's syndrome B. Down's syndrome
C. Achondroplasia D. TOF

860. **Picture frame vertebrae are seen typically in :**
A. Paget's disease B. Fluorosis
C. Ankylosing spondylitis D. Achondroplasia

861. **In Down's syndrome there are ------ ribs :**
A. 16 B. 18
C. 20 D. 22

862. **Rain drop lesions are seen in :**
A. Scurvy B. Thallasemia
C. Multiple myeloma D. Rickets

863. **Definite widening of the joints of hands and spine indicate :**
A. Gout B. Acromegaly
C. Hemophila D. Scleroderma

Ans. 854. B 855. D 856. D 857. A 858. A 859. B
860. A 861. D 862. C 863. B

864. **X-ray appearance of avascular necrosis before appearance of typical features :**
   A. Epiphyseal widening
   B. Increase in joint line
   C. Swelling of joint capsule
   D. Fixed deformity

865. **In Madeling deformity cardinal abnormality is :**
   A. Polydactyly
   B. Congenital absence of ulna
   C. Defective development of epiphysis of lower end of radius
   D. Synostosis of radius and ulna

866. **Periosteal reactions are not seen in :**
   A. Multiple myeloma
   B. Actinomycosis
   C. Infantile cortical hyperostosis
   D. Osteoid osteoma
   E. Syphilis

867. **The femur is fractured at birth at :**
   A. Upper one third B. Middle one third
   C. Lower one third D. Neck region

868. **Both knee joints show narrowing, subarticular cystic defects and deep, wide intercondylar fossae indicating probable :**
   A. Hemophilia B. Gout
   C. Rheumatoid arthritis D. Degenerative arthritis

869. **The cervical spine of a young adult showing several fused small joints bilaterally with underdeveloped vertebral bodies sharing narrowed intervertebral discs indicates probable childhood:**
   A. Trauma B. Septic arthritis
   C. Neurotropic disease D. Still's disease

870. **Cystic bone lesions with precocious sexual development and irregular pigmentation of the back indicate :**
   A. Gaucher's disease B. Neurofibromatosis
   C. Albright's syndrome D. Ollier's disease

Ans. 864. A 865. C 866. A 867. A 868. A 869. D 870. C

871. **Sacroiliitis is seen in the following, except :**
A. Whipple's disease B. Sarcoidosis
C. Reiter's syndrome D. Behcet's disease
E. Psoriasis

872. **Radiological evidence of secondaries in spine is evident when —— % of bone has been destroyed.**
A. 10 B. 30
C. 50 D. 80

873. **Not characteristic of Brodie's abscess is :**
A. Epiphyseal location
B. Sclerotic border
C. Chronic course
D. Localized radiant abscess in bone

874. **A multicystic process without bone reaction in the metaphysis of a long bone of a child is most likely :**
A. Bone infarct B. Tuberculosis
C. Osteogenesic sarcoma D. Pyogenic osteomyelitis

875. **Radiologically appreciable earliest sign of osteomyelitis is:**
A. Loss of muscle and fat planes
B. Periosteal reaction
C. Callus formation
D. Presence of sequestrum

876. **Increased density in the metaphyses of the long bones in children occurs in all, except :**
A. Scurvy B. Syphilis
C. Mercury poisoning D. Caffey's disease
E. Metaphyseal dysostosis

877. **Osteoblastic metastasis is most frequently seen in malignancy of :**
A. Lung B. Liver
C. Kidney D. Prostate

878. **All of the following causes increased bone density except :**
A. Fluorosis B. Osteopetrosis
C. Cushing's syndrome D. Prostate metastasis

879. **All of the following has decreased bone density except for :**
A. Hypophosphatasia B. Steroid therapy
C. Osteomalacia D. Hypervitaminosis-A

Ans. 871. B 872. C 873. A 874. B 875. B 876. D
877. D 878. C 879. D

880. Multiple Wormian bones can be seen in all, except :

A. Neonatal hypothyroidism

B. Down's syndrome

C. Fibrous dysplasia

D. Progeria

E. Normal babies

881. Incorrect about pathological fractures :

A. Are commonly transverse in long bones.

B. In Paget's disease, commonly occurs in the shaft of the femur.

C. Commonly occurs in the areas of chronic osteomyelitis.

D. Occurs in the subtrochanteric region of the femoral shaft.

E. Occurs as separation of the proximal femoral epiphysis in children with renal osteodystrophy.

882. Earliest bone metastasis can be detected by :

A. Compound tomography

B. Plain X-rays

C. Radio-isoscope bone scan

D. Tomography

883. The best X-ray view for the evaluation of a scaphoid fracture is :

A. Anteroposterior B. Lateral

C. Oblique D. Axial

884. "Tumbling blocks" appearance in an X-ray of the spine is seen in :

A. Sickle cell disease B. Neurosyphilis

C. Multiple myeloma D. Ankylosing spondylitis

885. In trisomy 18 syndrome, all are true, except :

A. Hypoplastic ribs are typical

B. The acetabular roof is flat

C. The first metacarpal is short

D. There is lumbar kyphoscoliosis

E. 'Rocker bottom' feet are characteristic

Ans. 880. C 881. C 882. C 883. C 884. C 885. B

886. **Jaccoud's arthritis occurs after the subsidence of severe bounds of :**
A. Rheumatic fever B. Crohn's disease
C. Amoebic colitis D. Acute glomerulonephritis
E. Ulcerative colitis

887. **Ossification may be commonly seen in ------- and ------.**
A. Mitral stenosis, lung bases
B. Mitral stenosis, lung apices
C. Mitral regurgitation, heart
D. Eisenmenger's complex, heart

888. **Looser's zone, osteosclerosis and subperiosteal erosion are seen in:**
A. Osteomalacia B. Renal osteodystrophy
C. Hyperparathyroidism D. Osteoporosis

889. **The bone most commonly involved in osteoarthritic change of the knee joint is :**
A. Femur
B. Patella
C. Fibula
D. All are involved at the same time

890. **A break in the Shenton's line is seen in :**
A. Down's syndrome
B. Congenital dislocation of hip
C. Cretinism
D. All of the above

891. **The break in spondylosis is at the :**
A. Superior articular process
B. Inferior articular process
C. Spinous process
D. Pars interarticularis

892. **Rib notching is seen in :**
A. Coarctation of aorta
B. Neurofibromatosis
C. Following Blalock-Taussig operation
D. All of the above

Ans. 886. A 887. A 888. B 889. B 890. B 891. D 892. D

893. Marginal posterior fracture passing through the radial articular surface is :

A. Smith's fracture B. Barton's fracture

C. Bennett's fracture D. Monteggia's fracture

894. Acro-osteolysis resorption of tips of the finger and toes is seen in :

A. Scleroderma B. Pyknodysostosis

C. Psoriasis D. All of the above

895. Which of the following does not describe chondroblastoma :

A. Non-calcifying

B. Eccentric

C. Epiphyseal location

D. Simulates giant cell tumour of bone

896. When a growing bone is traumatised there, may be a:

A. Outward depression of epiphysis

B. Shaftward depression of epiphysis

C. Shaft ward depression of metaphysis

D. All of the above

897. "Umbau Zones" are in all except :

A. Osteomalacia

B. Rickets

C. Osteogenesis imperfecta

D. Osteomyelitis

898. When fatigue fractures are multiple and symmetrical, the condition is known as :

A. Wax drippings B. Milkman's syndrome

C. Bone pearls D. None of the above

899. The Roentgen criteria for sesamoid fractures are all the following, except :

A. Irregular serrated line of division

B. Interrupted peripheral cortex

C. Multiplicity of fragments

D. Usual position

Ans. 893. B 894. D 895. A 896. C 897. C 898. B 899. D

900. **Commonest cause of punched out lesions in phalanges is:**
A. Enchondroma B. Chondrosarcoma
C. Aneurysmal bone cyst D. Multiple myeloma

901. **Calcification of the intervertebral disc is present in :**
A. Maple syrup urine disease
B. Homocystinuria
C. Ankylosing spondylitis
D. Achondroplasia

902. **Sun-rays appearance is seen in following, except :**
A. Multiple myeloma B. Sturge-Weber syndrome
C. Osteogenic sarcomas D. Meningioma

903. **Maisonneuve's sign indicates :**
A. Clavicle fracture
B. Colles' fracture
C. Smith fracture
D. Legg-Calve-Perthes disease

904. **Paget's disease of bone may be complicated by the following, except :**
A. Banana fracture
B. Pseudofracture
C. Basilar invigination
D. Severe neurological complications
E. Strengthening of bone as a result of periosteal addition

905. **Impacted fracture is found in :**
A. Neck of femur B. Neck of humerus
C. Lower end of radius D. All of the above

906. **Transverse process fracture of spine most often occurs at ----- region.**
A. Cervical B. Dorsal
C. Lumbar D. Sacral

907. **Cone shaped epiphyses in the phalanges can be seen in the following, except :**
A. After frost bite
B. As a normal variant
C. In cleidocranial dysostosis
D. In osteogenesis imperfecta

Ans. 900. A 901. C 902. B 903. B 904. E 905. C
906. C 907. D

908. Commonest site of spinal bifida is :

A. Cervical B. Dorsal

C. Lumbar D. Sacral

909. "Candle wax" appearance is seen in :

A. Osteogenesis imperfecta

B. Melorheostosis

C. Diaphyseal dysplasia

D. Exostosis

910. Radiologically appreciable earliest sign of osteomyelitis is :

A. Loss of muscles and fat planes

B. Periosteal reaction

C. Callus formation

D. Presence of sequestrum

911. Commonest site of fracture in osteogenesis imperfecta is :

A. Epiphysis B. Metaphysis

C. Diaphysis D. All of the above

912. All the following statements are true about Fibrous Dysplasia except for :

A. Ground-glass appearance of bone

B. Shepherd-Crook's appearance of femur

C. Commoner in females

D. Lesions are classically bilateral

913. Normal metacarpal index is :

A. Less than 5.4 B. 5.4 to 7.9

C. 8.4 to 10.4 D. More than 10.4

914. Metacarpal index is increased in the case of :

A. Down's syndrome B. Marfan's syndrome

C. Turner's syndrome D. Jeene's disease

915. Which of the following radio isotopes is used orally for treating a case of carcinoma presents with secondaries in bone :

A. Strontium B. Co60

C. Cs D. Ra

916. Earliest sign in rheumatoid arthritis is :

A. Decreased joint space

B. Periarticular ssteoporosis

C. Periarticular soft tissue swelling

D. Reduced joint space

Ans. 908. C 909. B 910. A 911. C 912. D 913. B
914. B 915. A 916. B

917. 'Fat-pad-sign' may be present in fracture of lateral epicondyle of salter type----injury.
A. I B. II
C. III D. V

918. Avulsion fracture is most common in ------ metatarsal.
A. I B. II
C. III D. IV

919. Early radiological sign of caries spine is :
A. Wedging of vertebra
B. Syndesmophyte formation
C. Formation of paravertebral abscess
D. Decreased joint space

920. Commonest type of spinal TB is :
A. Anterior B. Posterior
C. Central D. Paradiscal
E. All of the above

921. Radiological features of rickets are all, except :
A. Narrowing and loss of zone of provisional calcification is earliest sign.
B. Metaphyseal margin becomes indistinct.
C. Frayed appearance.
D. Splaying and cupping of metaphyseal markings.
E. After one year of treatment only, recovery starts in X-rays.

922. In bony metastasis, primary should be looked for in all, except :
A. Prostate B. Thyroid
C. Stomach D. Bronchus

923. Multiple osteolytic lesions in a 2 years, child in skull and long bones are seen in :
A. Neuroblastoma B. Histiocytosis
C. Thalassemia major D. Wilms tumor

924. Flask shaped femur is seen in all, except :
A. Osteomalacia B. Osteopetrosis
C. Gaucher's disease D. Thalassemia

Ans. 917. B 918. D 919. D 920. D 921. E 922. C
923. A 924. A

925. **Saw tooth metaphysis are seen in :**
A. Acromegaly B. Hyperparathyroidism
C. Congenital syphilis D. Ochronosis

926. **Syndactyly is seen in all of the following, except :**
A. Laurence Moon Biedel disease
B. Apert's syndrome
C. Trisomy-13
D. Madelung deformity

927. **Commonest fatal skeletal dysplasia of new-born is :**
A. Osteogenesis imperfecta type-II
B. Thanatophoric dwarfism
C. Camptomelic dwarfism
D. Homozygous form of achondroplasia

Match the X-ray land marks of foetal development with the period (Ques. 1037 to 1041):
A. 32 weeks B. 36 weeks
C. 24 weeks D. 12 weeks
E. 38 weeks

928. **Distal femoral epiphysis**
929. **Foetal fat line**
930. **Calcaneous**
931. **Proximal tibial epiphysis**
932. **Spine and skull**

933. **Piano key sign is seen in :**
A. Osteoarthritis
B. Rheumatoid arthritis
C. Ankylosing spondylitis
D. Reiter's syndrome

934. **In multiple myeloma, the radiologically differentiating manifestation is commonly seen in :**
A. Skull B. Vertebra
C. Ribs D. Pelvis

935. **Splaying and cupping of the metaphysis is seen in :**
A. Rickets B. Scurvy
C. Paget's disease D. Lead poisoning

Ans.	925. C	926. B	927. B	928. B	929. A	930. C
	931. E	932. D	933. B	934. B	935. A	

936. Radiological manifestation of acute osteomyelitis within first 8 days is :
A. Cystic swelling
B. Sequestrum
C. Subperiosteal new bone
D. Soft tissue swelling

937. Commonest cause of epiphyseal thickening in children is:
A. Congenital syphilis
B. Rickets
C. Scurvy
D. Osteochondrodystrophy

938. 76-years-old man presents with lytic lesions in the vertebra. X-ray skull showed multiple punched-out lesions. The most likely diagnosis is :
A. Multiple myeloma B. Hyperparathyroidism
C. Metastasis D. Osteomalacia

939. Posterior iliac horn is seen in :
A. Nail patella syndrome B. Ankylosing spondylitis
C. Hurler's syndrome D. Marfan's syndrome

940. Chondrocalcinosis is seen in :
A. Hyperthyroidism B. Ochronosis
C. Hypoparathyroidism D. Hypervitaminosis-D

941. In bone scan, hot spots are seen in all, except :
A. Osteoblastic metastasis
B. Multiple myeloma
C. Osteomyelitis
D. Bony lesions of hyperparathyroidism

942. Mutton-leg like gross appearance is seen in :
A. Osteosarcoma B. Osteoclastoma
C. Chondrosarcoma D. Ewing's sarcoma

943. Linear accelerator provide :
A. Both electrons & X-rays
B. Only electrons
C. Protons
D. Electromagnetic rays

Ans. 936. D 937. B 938. A 939. A 940. B 941. B
942. A 943. A

944. Which of the following is a recognized X-ray feature of rheumatoid arthritis :
A. Juxta-articular osteosclerosis
B. Sacrolitis
C. Bone-erosions
D. Peri-articular calcification

945. Fraying and cupping of metaphysis of long bones in an child does not occur in which of the following :
A. Rickets
B. Lead poisoning
C. Metaphyseal dysplasia
D. Hypophosphatasia

946. The gold standard for the diagnosis of osteoporosis is :
A. Dual energy X-ray absorptiometry
B. Single energy X-ray absorptiometry
C. Ultrasound
D. Quantitative computed tomography

947. Calcification of posterior spinal ligament is best diagnosed by :
A. MRI
B. CT
C. X-ray
D. USG

948. Which of the following is not a cause of generalized increase in bone density in adult :
A. Myelosclerosis
B. Renal osteodystrophy
C. Fluorosis
D. Caffey's diseases

Ans. 944. C 945. D 946. A 947. B 948. D